NUTRITIONAL THERAPY

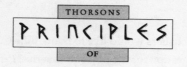

NUTRITIONAL THERAPY

LINDA LAZARIDES

Thorsons
An Imprint of HarperCollinsPublishers

The publishers would like to thank Jillie Collings
for her suggestion for the title of this series, *Principles of...*

Thorsons
An Imprint of HarperCollins*Publishers*
77–85 Fulham Palace Road,
Hammersmith, London W6 8JB
1160 Battery Sreet
San Francisco, California 94111–1213

Published by Thorsons 1996

3 5 7 9 10 8 6 4

Linda Lazarides assert the moral right to
be identified as the authors of this work

A catalogue record for this book
is available from the British Library

ISBN 0 7225 3285 7

Printed and bound in Great Britain by
Caledonian International Book Manufacturing Ltd, Glasgow

CONTENTS

INTRODUCTION

Margaret had been trying to lose weight for eight years when she first consulted me. She was five feet three inches tall, and weighed eleven and a half stone, but no matter what she did the weight wouldn't come off. She really starved herself, eating no breakfast and no lunch, just a green salad and a sardine or a tablespoon of cottage cheese in the evenings, with a teaspoon of sunflower seeds, followed by an apple or tangerine. She never ate puddings, sweets or chocolates, never added sugar to anything, and never ate bread, biscuits, cakes or pastry, potatoes, fried food, butter or margarine. Margaret got up at 6 am to ensure that she got in half an hour's jogging every morning before going to work.

Margaret's doctor didn't believe that she was dieting. He thought that she was inventing all this and secretly stuffing herself with junk food. He referred her to a dietitian, who gave her a 1000-calorie a day diet. Margaret gained weight when she followed the diet. She was in despair by the time she consulted me.

Nutritional therapy is a form of complementary medicine. It should never be confused with dietetics or 'nutrition'. There are two vital differences between these disciplines. A nutritional therapist carries out a diagnostic procedure and works towards a therapeutic goal. In other words, he or she tries to answer the questions 'what is making this person ill?' and 'what can I do to get them better?' A dietitian's job, on the other hand, is to carry out a doctor's instructions and to advise on healthy eating in accordance with official guidelines. The doctor makes the diagnosis (anaemia, irritable bowel syndrome and so on) and refers the patient to a dietitian for a diet high in iron or a high-fibre diet. Some dietitians work in hospitals, for instance giving patients with severe liver or kidney disease diets to manage these conditions, that is to say diets to help them cope with the disease.

Nutritional therapists rarely see such seriously ill people. They hope that people will come to them when the first small symptoms begin and there is a better chance of reversing them. Unfortunately a trip to the doctor at this stage may result in negative tests and a reassurance that nothing is wrong. So no action is taken and people who are tired all the time, or who have bad skin, digestive problems, headaches or female complaints frequently try instead to ignore their symptoms because they don't want to be thought of as time wasters.

It is probably true in a lot of cases that you would be wasting your doctor's time if you continue to complain about problems like these after being told that nothing is wrong. Your doctor is looking for an identifiable disease, for which the textbooks specify a definite treatment, usually involving drugs or surgery.

In complementary medicine we take small symptoms as a sign that the body's health is for some reason under assault. There can be many different reasons for this assault, including stress, poor eating habits, wear and tear, a slow build-up of toxic waste substances, allergy or intolerance to certain foods or environmental factors, chronic infections, self-abuse with excess alcohol, caffeine or other drugs, poor alignment of bones or joints leading to pressure on blood vessels, nerves or spinal cord, or poor digestion leading to nutritional deficiencies. Some branches of complementary medicine see ill- health as a disturbance to the body's electrical or 'life force' energy.

Fortunately Margaret was so desperate to find out what was wrong with her that she took the plunge of seeking an alternative therapist. So I tried to diagnose what made Margaret put on weight so easily.

There were several different possible causes. Firstly, her thyroid gland might be underfunctioning. Although the thyroid test which her doctor had carried out was normal, it might have been at the lower end of normal, verging on the hypothyroid. Standard thyroid tests are thought to be a little insensitive, and not always guaranteed to reveal borderline hypothyroidism. Since an underfunctioning thyroid often means a reduced metabolic rate (the thyroid gland governs the metabolism), Margaret just might not be able to burn up even 1,000 calories a day, and was turning some of them into fat instead.

Secondly, Margaret might have been retaining fluid, and her excess weight might not be body fat but water. Fluid retention can be caused by protein deficiency, vitamin or mineral deficiency, allergy, by certain drugs, or by an excess of yin (a Chinese term) in the body. Yin refers to a type of energy in oriental medicine, inherent in foods or conditions of the body that can be described as cold, watery or loose. It is the opposite of yang, which is the energy inherent in foods or conditions of the body that can be described as hot, dry or dense.

Since Margaret's problem did not resolve when she ate a diet higher in protein, it was unlikely that the problem was protein-related. She was also taking vitamin and mineral supplements, so a deficiency of these could not be the cause either. She was not eating any common food allergens, and had none of the usual allergic symptoms like headaches, bowel upsets or skin rashes, so I did not believe that the problem was allergy-related. I asked Margaret whether she felt the cold easily, and she confirmed that she did. A temperature test carried out at home first thing in the morning confirmed that her resting body temperature was quite low, and this tended to suggest both an underfunctioning thyroid gland and an excess of yin.

I was very reluctant to allow Margaret to continue eating only one meal a day. Her food intake was so small that she was in danger of not getting adequate amounts of other nutrients. But Margaret was so afraid of putting on weight that she was very reluctant to eat more. Eventually we compromised, with an agreement that Margaret would eat soup at lunchtime and a meal in the evening. The soup was to be made from lentils, onions, carrots and miso (a nutritious Japanese broth available from health food shops). In the evening she was to have a small serving of brown rice, with some fish and cooked vegetables.

I increased Margaret's intake of magnesium, iron, vitamin B_6 and zinc, and also prescribed GLA (from evening primrose oil) since some minor symptoms such as severely flaking fingernails suggested she was deficient. Although it is a common belief that iodine supplements in the form of kelp help to 'boost' the thyroid gland, I did not prescribe kelp tablets: a daily fish intake together with the iodine included in multiminerals ensures a more than adequate intake. Excessive iodine can be detrimental to the thyroid gland.

We waited to see what the new diet and supplements would do. After two weeks there were no real changes yet but Margaret was delighted that her new diet had not made her put on weight although she was eating three times her previous calorie intake. After four weeks Margaret came in beaming from ear to ear. She had lost 4 lb. She was also feeling warmer and more energetic and told me that she hadn't realized how little energy she'd had before. An unexpected bonus was the return of her sex drive, which had been very low for some years. Margaret went on to lose another half stone before I discharged her from my care, and she felt like a new woman.

HOW DID IT WORK?

Margaret's story is a very good illustration of the principles of nutritional therapy. Firstly, I took Margaret seriously and did not trivialize her problem or accuse her of lying as all others had done. I was willing to look for a solution for her. By getting to know her health history, diet history and every detail of her present state of health, from fingernail condition to energy levels, it was possible to apply knowledge of simple nutritional biochemistry and physiology to her individual case. Ancient principles of medicine were also extremely important. In both Western herbalism and oriental medicine it is accepted that a condition of the body can be influenced by both the chemistry and the physics of plants and other foods. So in the West we give the herb comfrey to people with broken bones because it contains tissue-building nutrients, and we might also give the herb plantain to pass on its quality of resilience: plaintain quickly springs back to shape if crushed. In oriental medicine it is accepted that an excess consumption of cold wet foods can lead to a cold, water-logged body therefore we would aim to treat this condition with foods that have the opposite physical quality.

It was a simple matter to change Margaret from raw salads and cold fish to hot lentil soup, warm fish and cooked rice and vegetables. Lentils and rice are compact, dense and dry before cooking, properties which we were aiming to encourage in Margaret's body to drive out the excess fluid.

There are those who prefer to explain away results like

Margaret's. Typical comments might be: 'The shape and size of foods, and whether they are hot or cold cannot possibly affect body weight so the patient must have been lying about her original diet.'

Explaining things away is of course easy, but it is not productive.

THE UNIQUENESS PRINCIPLE

Margaret's case also illustrates another principle, which is at the core of the difference between orthodox and complementary medicine. If the foods which I had prescribed for Margaret (lentil soup, fish, rice and cooked vegetables) are so special, and can cause weight loss regardless of calorie content, then (say conventional scientists) they should work for everyone, and a clinical trial should be able to prove it.

Complementary medicine practitioners always come up against this problem when trying to communicate with those who are untrained in our system of medicine. Western medicine says that if a treatment is to be proven valid, it should work on a significant percentage of people. But what people? If you simply take a group of people with the same symptoms and give them all the same treatment, that's a bit like giving all broken-down TV sets the same new spare part in the hope of restoring the picture.

The complementary medicine practitioner is a bit like a professional TV repair man. He or she carries out a diagnostic procedure not to name the symptoms but to try to identify the cause of the malfunction before prescribing a treatment. So just as 100 different TV sets may need 100 different spare parts even though the symptoms are the same, people should have individualized treatments according to the cause of their illness. After all (as some wise person said) the human body can only suffer from a limited number of symptoms, but there are an infinite number of possible causes!

Margaret's Western diagnosis was that she was overweight. My diagnosis was that she was cold and overly 'yin', with a slow metabolism and an essential fatty acid deficiency, and was probably retaining fluid. Give me 50 people all exactly like this and Margaret's diet would very likely have similar effects on all of them. But don't expect me to use the diet on 50 people simply diagnosed as 'overweight'!

A BRIEF HISTORY OF NUTRITIONAL THERAPY

Nutritional therapy is probably the oldest form of medicine in existence. From the Jewish tradition of feeding chicken soup to the sick, to the discovery that lemons (not limes as most people think – lime is in fact an old word for lemon) could treat scurvy, nutritional therapy is familiar to all of us in one form or another. Sometimes nutritional therapy considerably overlaps with herbal medicine. When plants are given for their therapeutic value, do they work because they are nourishing the body, restoring the raw materials which it needs to perform its many tasks? Or do they work as medicines, exogenous substances which normally have no physiological role in the body but can alter its function? We don't know but there is no doubt that many plants, whether herbal medicines or foods, play a very useful role in nutritional therapy.

In the West, nutritional therapy was until recently known primarily as part of the system referred to as 'naturopathy' which began in the late nineteenth and early twentieth centuries. During this era fashionable medical treatments often used dangerous heavy metals like mercury and arsenic to treat diseases. The naturopathy movement, led by figures like Vincent Priessnitz, Sebastian Kneipp and J.H. Kellogg was a reaction against this. Its members believed that it was more effective to treat disease with natural methods like diets and fasting to eliminate toxins and nourish the body, thus stimulating the body's own natural self-healing ability.

The early naturopaths believed that food should be as close to nature as possible, and preferably raw. Mainstream naturopathy has now moderated its views somewhat, and raw food is no longer advocated for everyone. (Those who continue to adhere to a raw food philosophy are now called 'natural hygienists'.)

Nutritional therapy as we now know it was born from three parents: the naturopathy movement, and the more recent nutritional medicine and allergy and environmental medicine movements, which were themselves only born in the latter half of the twentieth century.

NUTRITIONAL MEDICINE

Some of the eminent figures in the early nutritional medicine movement were Abram Hoffer, Roger Williams, Irwin Stone and Frederick Klenner. These were followed by other outstanding figures such as Linus Pauling and Carl Pfeiffer, and more recently Jeffrey Bland and Stephen Davies – all doctors and scientists involved in the treatment of disease primarily by nutritional means.

Hoffer, an eminent psychiatrist, was interested in the possible beneficial effects of large doses of nutrients against schizophrenia. This was soon after the discovery that the mystery disease pellagra, which was originally thought to be a form of mental illness and was practically indistinguishable from schizophrenia, could be cured with large doses of niacin (vitamin B_3) and was simply a nutritional deficiency disease. Hoffer's team used large doses of vitamin B_3 and vitamin C to inhibit the formation of adrenochrome, a form of oxidized adrenaline which is found in high levels in schizophrenics. Although the results of his research were considered by others to be inconclusive, he did have much success and his work continues today. Much similar research was going on at the time. Many vitamins had only just been discovered, and investigations of their potential as drugs were quite fashionable until new wonder drugs like cortisone came on the scene. Thousands of studies into the potential benefits of increased amounts of vitamins and minerals against hundreds of diseases can be found in the medical literature of the 1950s.

In the USA in particular, this research was not forgotten even when vitamins were no longer fashionable treatments. Many doctors, such as Frederick Klenner, who were treating their patients with dietary supplements, felt certain that if patients responded to these measures then they were suffering from subclinical nutritional deficiencies and no amount of any wonder drug could take the place of the nutrients they needed. What kept reaffirming their belief in a nutritional approach was the fact that such a large proportion of their patients seemed to benefit from it. Nutritional deficiencies must indeed be widespread – far more common than is generally believed.

And there was vitamin C. Irwin Stone, a member of the nutritional medicine movement and a great enthusiast of the benefits of vitamin C therapy, collated the results of thousands of research studies and came to the conclusion that vitamin C supplementation had such widespread benefits that this could only be explained by endemic deficiency – a deficiency of the vitamin in the whole human race. This theory may not be as outlandish as it sounds. Man is one of only a tiny handful of species among mammals which cannot manufacture their own vitamin C from glucose, in the liver. Humans in fact have a genetic defect: we are missing the final enzyme in the manufacturing process, which virtually all other mammals have.

Linus Pauling, twice a Nobel Prize laureate and one of the most eminent scientists of his time, became fascinated by Stone's work in the early 1970s, and began to champion the cause of vitamin C therapy. Pauling and Stone estimated that an animal the size of a human would be able to make about 18 grams a day of vitamin C in its liver (more if it was ill or under stress).

On the basis of the research, Pauling was particularly fascinated by vitamin C's potential as a treatment for the common cold and for cancer. Taking the daily quantities synthesized by animals as a guideline for human needs, he urged researchers to use dosages for humans in grams rather than in milligrams, but they rarely did so. This was frustrating for Pauling and his colleagues, since the use of low dosages would invariably fail to confirm the full value of the treatment. Unfortunately such failure was construed by others as confirmation that vitamin C itself was a worthless treatment.

In the late 1970s Pauling teamed up with a Scottish physician Ewan Cameron to treat terminal cancer patients with ten grams a day of vitamin C at the Vale of Leven hospital. Although the results of the trial were very encouraging, with several of the patients surviving for many years after the dates predicted for their death, most of the medical establishment resisted Cameron and Pauling's efforts to repeat the study using larger numbers of patients, and the whole subject became extremely controversial.

By the early 1980s nutritional medicine, which Pauling, writer Adelle Davis and others had helped to popularize, was spreading from the USA to the United Kingdom and other parts of the world, where the public eagerly seized on the information. It was around this time that the nutritional therapy movement was born in the UK. Here it developed separately from the current naturopathic movement which never really took it fully on board. In the USA and Australia, naturopathic colleges like the Bastyr College did tend to incorporate the new principles of nutritional therapy, and by the late 1980s the use of vitamin supplements and healthy diets was enormously fashionable, with the public if not with the medical profession. In the UK three schools specializing in the teaching of nutritional therapy had opened, and several hundred specialist practitioners were now in practice.

ALLERGY AND ENVIRONMENTAL MEDICINE

The clinical ecology movement, which was later to become known as the allergy and environmental medicine movement, began in the 1940s, also in the USA. Its founding father is generally considered to be allergist Theron Randolph MD, who believed that up to 30 per cent of all people who consult a doctor have symptoms partially or wholly due to food or environmental allergies. Dr Randolph wrote copiously to publicize his methods, which were generally rejected by orthodox doctors. Other famous figures in the environmental medicine movement who followed Dr Randolph were Richard Mackarness, Bill Rae (USA) and Jean Monro (UK).

The environmental medicine and nutritional medicine movements were natural team-mates, and most doctors who became interested in one soon discovered the other. Schools training nutritional therapists in the UK also incorporated allergy investigations into their programmes, and it is routine for the nutritional therapist to carry out such investigations with their patients.

It is estimated that more than 60,000 chemicals are now in current production, and another 6,000 come on the market every year. Environmental medicine specialists carry out laboratory investigations to measure levels of common pollutants in the body, and use nutritional regimes to help the body eliminate them. By the mid-1990s the blending of the two disciplines was becoming highly sophisticated, with experts like Dr Jeffrey Bland and Bill Rae in particular helping to unite the scientific element of the natural health movement and keep it, as well as the lay practitioners, up to date with the latest research into pollutant damage and detoxification.

And so nutritional therapy was born. As yet its main stronghold is still the English-speaking world. Almost universally rejected by the medical establishment throughout the world, its spread and propagation rely on lay practitioners and laws that allow the public to buy dietary supplements freely at the levels needed for therapeutic use. Unfortunately although the naturopathic movement is still strong in Europe, laws in most Western European countries do not permit the free sale of dietary supplements at the dosages found in the UK, North America and Australia. And in many of these countries it is illegal to practise any form of medicine unless you are a doctor. There are worries that the European Commission will decide to legislate on dietary supplements and natural medicine, which would result in the certain destruction of the freedom currently experienced in the UK and Holland. This is because EC legislation is always based on the majority view of the Council of Ministers, which is in turn based on the national laws of the various countries. Countries with minority views simply have to fall into line.

WHAT IS NUTRITIONAL THERAPY?

A clear distinction has to be drawn between nutritional therapy proper and self-help using diet and supplements. Nutritional therapy requires a specialist practitioner with training in physiology, biochemistry and pathology as well as naturopathic techniques, nutrition and the principles of environmental medicine. Nutritional therapy also requires a diagnostic procedure, which uses this extensive knowledge to determine an individual's possible nutritional needs. On its own a doctor's diagnosis is not usually of very much help in designing natural health programmes.

To take an example, while some studies have shown that evening primrose oil is beneficial for a doctor's diagnosis of eczema, you may very well find that your eczema does not improve very much when you try taking evening primrose oil. Similarly magnesium supplementation has been found to lower blood pressure in some clinical trials, but books containing this information probably won't mention the other clinical trials where magnesium didn't work.

The fact is, only allopathic medicines are designed for use with orthodox medical diagnoses. Evening primrose oil is not a medicine, it is a nutritional product, and as such it can only treat deficiencies of the nutrients it contains, in this case gamma linolenic acid or GLA. Exactly the same applies to magnesium and other nutrients.

I have known many people who believed that they were capable of diagnosing and treating themselves on the basis of information obtained from books. Every practitioner's patients have already tried to treat themselves, and if they had been successful they would not be consulting the practitioner. In attempting to self-treat there is a very real danger that the conclusions reached may be superficial, leading the patient completely off the right track and sometimes to a dangerously inadequate diet. There is also the unfortunate possibility that unsuccessful self-treatment may lead to disillusionment with the therapy when what was needed was simply proper professional advice.

One of the problems that can occur with books is bias. Does the book give you the full story? For instance it may tell you that B vitamin deficiency causes fatigue, but does it explain *all* the possible causes of fatigue, which can range from a poor diet to worm or parasite infestations? And if you find yourself identifying with a long list of B vitamin deficiency symptoms does the book caution you that all these symptoms can also be explained by something else?

SELF-DIAGNOSIS CAN BE MISLEADING

One of my patients (let's call him Jeremy) was suffering from severe digestive problems. He felt sick all the time, and had a constant pain in his tummy. After eating he would have burning sensations in the stomach. Jeremy's doctor could find nothing wrong with him, gave him antacids (which didn't stop the problem) and a course of steroid drugs to help him put on weight. Jeremy didn't take these for long because of unpleasant side effects and worries about the dangers of such drugs.

Jeremy was determined to find the answer to his health problems somehow, and began a quest on the bookshelves of his local health food shop. He tried food combining (a system of avoiding eating starch and protein in the same meal), which seemed to help a bit. Then he found another book which advised him to eat nothing except fruit until lunch-time. The third book was about candidiasis, which he convinced himself that he suffered from, and so stopped eating all fruit and sweet foods. Since his breakfast had been fruit, he was reduced to two meals a day. Still not feeling better he thought that perhaps raw food was the answer, as it seemed to be all that was left to try, and he progressed to eating nothing but raw food. I also gained the impression that, perhaps subconsciously, Jeremy became attached to this diet because it was so strict and difficult. He had somehow associated healthy eating with deprivation and believed that the more he deprived himself the more good he was doing himself.

As you can imagine, by now Jeremy, on only two meals a day consisting of raw vegetables and salad, was rapidly losing weight. Although his height was five feet nine, he dropped to seven and a half stone and, feeling very ill, returned to his doctor, who diagnosed him as anorexic until he realised what was going on. Of course Jeremy was simply trying to find the diet that would cure him, believing very firmly that nutrition was the answer to his health problems.

On his doctor's advice, Jeremy gave up trying to find the perfect diet for a while, and reverted to a high-fat, high-sugar diet. In many ways he felt better eating a lot of junk food, probably because he was no longer dangerously underweight, but his digestive problems did not go away.

By the time Jeremy first consulted me, his weight was normal. His skin was very bad, with eczema-like rashes, his self-image appalling, and his confidence at a very low ebb. It became clear very soon that Jeremy's tummy pain and nausea were coming from his liver, which was tender to the touch, and his gall bladder. When the gall bladder is congested or contains stones, it hurts when fatty food is consumed, because fat in the diet stimulates the gall bladder to contract and release its contents. The contraction may be quite painful and cause painful spasms in the muscles around that area, as well as referred pain (pain originating from a site other than where it is felt) elsewhere in the body.

I was fairly sure that what seemed to be an over-acid condition of the stomach was probably the opposite. Jeremy's digestion was very poor. He suffered from severe flatulence if he attempted to eat vegetables, and they would often emerge practically undigested in his stools. Acid burning can be caused by a delayed production of stomach acid as well as by an excess. When stomach acid production is delayed, the stomach contents may be already in the duodenum by the time the acid is produced. Then the stomach burns because there is no food to buffer it.

The next stage of digestion, which requires enzymes produced by the pancreas and small intestine, cannot take place properly unless the food leaving the stomach has a low (acidic) pH. This is because the presence of acid is needed to stimulate the production of bicarbonate by the liver and pancreas. In turn the bicarbonate makes the gut contents more alkaline, and this acts as a trigger for the release of digestive enzymes.

So what Jeremy needed was a hydrochloric acid supplement and the herb gentian (which stimulates the digestion) to ensure that his food would be acidic enough to trigger off the rest of the digestive process. He also needed supplements of the fatty acids EPA and GLA, having developed severe deficiencies of these due to his digestive difficulties. (His skin rash and dandruff were almost certainly caused by malabsorption of these nutrients.) Jeremy also needed a diet low in saturated fat because his nausea and pain were liver-related and caused by the large amount of saturated fat in his diet. The essential fat that he needed in his diet could be provided by wholegrains like brown rice and porridge oats, as well as a little extra virgin olive oil, which doesn't seem to cause liver spasms like other forms of fat. Another important aspect of treatment was to give Jeremy herbs to soothe his liver and gall bladder, and help them to decongest as quickly as possible.

This treatment programme was very different from what Jeremy had tried to administer himself. It made an enormous difference to Jeremy's health, and though his digestion remained sensitive (due to his nervous anxiety more than anything else), his skin improved, he digested his food better and the liver-related pain and nausea (which had greatly added to his anxiety) gradually got better.

A LITTLE KNOWLEDGE CAN BE TOO SUPERFICIAL

In Jeremy's case there was no doctor's diagnosis, but the same problems apply to self-treatment when a diagnosis *has* been made. Let's take high blood pressure as an example. It seems simple enough, the books all advise you to lose weight, eat oily fish, eat lots of soluble fibre and stop eating salt. The authors make a lot of money from giving this advice, which is based on research studies using these techniques on people with high blood pressure.

But what if it doesn't work? How sad it would be if you had to take drugs for your blood pressure for the rest of your life when an investigation by a nutritional therapist might have given you a better chance of finding an alternative answer. There are in fact a number of possible factors involved in high

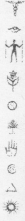

blood pressure. Giving everybody the same regime doesn't take this into account.

High blood pressure means that excessive amounts of pressure are being exerted on the walls of your arteries as your blood is pumped through them by your heart. You can create a similar effect if you try to turn on a high-pressure tap attached to a very thin hosepipe. The more water tries to get through, the greater the pressure that is exerted on the wall of the hosepipe. So giving blood will temporarily reduce your blood pressure; there is simply less to be pumped around. However giving blood is not a long-term solution!

Excessive thickness or stickiness of the blood can also increase the pressure. So can excessive fluid, as in the case of water retention. This is why diuretics are often prescribed by doctors – as long as you keep taking them they reduce the overall amount of fluid in your body.

Healthy vessel walls should be elastic and able to give a little when under pressure. On the other hand excessive rigidity or tension of the artery walls can increase the blood pressure.

Deposits of cholesterol which coat the artery walls can also increase the blood pressure. Their lumen (internal diameter) simply becomes smaller due to the deposits, making the flow more difficult.

The nutritional therapist will certainly assume that your blood may be too sticky, and, if you are not on anticoagulant drugs, may ask you to eat oily fish and/or take fish oil and vitamin E supplements because these help to thin the blood. But he or she will want to know answers to a number of questions before coming up with a regime for you.

For instance, do you drink a lot of coffee? Coffee consumption is linked with increased blood pressure and also causes a loss of precious minerals like magnesium through the urine by making you urinate more. Many people eat a very magnesium-poor diet. Using a lot of milk and dairy produce in particular can damage your magnesium status since they contain large amounts of calcium. Calcium competes with magnesium for absorption sites in the body. It is now becoming widely accepted that magnesium deficiency is associated with spasms and increased rigidity of the artery walls, which in turn can raise blood pressure. What is not widely accepted is that mild magnesium deficiency is a relatively common phenomenon.

How about your sugar consumption? Every time you eat sugar, you lose some of the trace element chromium in your urine. A chromium deficiency has also been linked with cardiovascular problems.

If your high blood pressure is also associated with swelling of your ankles or joints, pre-menstrual bloating, or fluid retention, then it may be due to an excess of fluid. The most common causes of a fluid build-up are probably kidney dysfunction or food allergy/intolerance. A nutritional therapist will want to find out if you are an allergic type, and will ask you if you also suffer from joint pains, headaches, hay fever, eczema, irritable bowel syndrome or sinusitus. If so, the therapist may well ask you to exclude certain foods with allergenic (allergy-causing) potential from your diet to see if the fluid is lost and the blood pressure accordingly reduced.

As far as cholesterol deposits in arteries are concerned, there is a lot more to combating this than eating a high-fibre diet. Certainly soluble fibre will help to prevent you reabsorbing the bile acids in your intestine, which are reconverted to cholesterol in the liver. But your liver itself may be faulty. Most of the cholesterol in your body does not come from your diet but is produced by your liver. The nutritional therapist will want to do some maintenance work on your liver with herbs and nutrients like lecithin to help it eliminate excess fat and function more efficiently.

And finally what about the research that never reaches the eminent medical journals that most doctors read? Two nutrients, vitamin C and the amino acid L-lysine, have the ability to latch on to cholesterol and slowly carry it away from sites where it has been deposited. Very large amounts of these nutrients are needed for this purpose, amounting to several grams a day. Cases of severe, almost terminal, angina (a condition involving a very serious build-up of cholesterol deposits in the coronary artery of the heart) have been completely reversed using this procedure.

WHO NEEDS NUTRITIONAL THERAPY?

C hoosing the right therapy is often a problem in complementary medicine. There are no research studies to say that therapy x is better than therapy y for arthritis/angina/eczema etc. Some choices are more obvious, like seeing an osteopath for back pain, but even then how do you know whether an osteopath, chiropractor or applied kinesiologist would be the best choice?

Professional practitioner associations sometimes ask their therapists to offer brief preliminary consultations at low cost or no charge to people who just want to know how likely the therapy is to benefit them. The nutritional therapist will use this opportunity to ask questions designed to identify the possible presence of food allergy or intolerance, toxic overload or nutritional deficiencies. If any of these are thought to be present, then, whatever their health problem, the client has a good chance of feeling better once a tailor-made programme has been developed.

This is not to say that all illnesses will be cured outright. If you suffer from cancer, rheumatoid arthritis, multiple sclerosis or any other serious disease it is important to deal with allergies, deficiencies and toxic overload since these undermine your body's strength and ability to fight illness, but the final outcome depends on your individual constitution and other factors such as emotional stress, physical stress, geopathic stress, electromagnetic fields, genetic inheritance and even climate. Ideally a therapist would want to work on as many of these factors as possible to aid the body in its fight against the disease.

IMPROVING EFFICIENCY AND FUNCTION

Many people ask, 'What's the point of looking for allergies when what I've got is cancer or multiple sclerosis?' It is important to remember that a sick person's body never stops fighting a disease. Often it wins the battle, as when you recover from a cold or the flu. But sometimes its defences are overwhelmed, and a chronic or degenerative illness sets in. To understand how complementary medicine works you need to bear in mind that the presence of an illness requires two conditions: (a) A disease process, and (b) The failure of the body to resist that process.

If we can work on (a), ascertaining and eliminating the cause(s) of a disease process, such as an infectious micro-organism, then we can cure the disease outright. If there is no known cause for the disease process, or no effective means of combating it directly, we can combat it indirectly by working on (b), generally helping the body to function more efficiently and therefore to fight illness more efficiently. As most of us in the nutritional therapy movement know from experience, the efficiency of most people's bodies can be improved by removing what is stressing them. There can be nothing more stressful for it to deal with than a deficiency of raw materials (nutrients), an excess of toxic waste substances and the presence of allergies, which the body must also summon up the energy to fight, alongside the disease process. All these problems are far more common than most people realize.

Another question which people ask is: 'I would know if I was allergic or if I had nutritional deficiencies. So why should I bother with seeing a practitioner?' I would like to answer this by describing my own case.

I grew up in the 1960s, when nutrition was still a relatively young science. My father, who worked in the pathology lab of a hospital, was interested in nutrition and particularly in the fact that it was now 'proved' to be an old wives' tale that we should all be getting lots of vitamins and minerals in our diet. In fact he detested vegetables and sought excuses in textbooks not to eat them. He found much learned material to support his cause, and would frequently quote it at home. 'We need such minute amounts of vitamins and minerals,' he would say, 'that as long as we eat some first-class protein (animal protein) every day, we can eat anything we like the rest of the time.' My mother dutifully cooked us meat and potatoes every day. We also had eggs, milk and white bread. There was rarely any fruit. By the time I reached puberty I was suffering from a wide range of minor symptoms.

The outside of my upper arms and legs were covered in what is known as 'toad skin' or hyperkeratosis pilaris, little bumps centred on hair follicles. I also had red, itchy patches around my eyebrows and nostrils. I could not sleep at night. I would lie awake tossing and turning until the early hours and wake up feeling very groggy the next day. But if I slept for too long I would develop a headache. I also had a headache if I didn't sleep enough.

The worst problem was intestinal wind and bloating, more or less constant and sometimes painful. Needless to say, I was also very constipated, perhaps managing a small bowel motion once a week. Although reasonably energetic, I didn't seem to

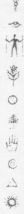

PRINCIPLES OF NUTRITIONAL THERAPY

have as much stamina as other children of my age. I got out of breath very easily. Sometimes I suffered from stitching pains in my heart, which stopped my breath. Menstruation was excruciatingly painful.

None of this was too serious, and I was considered a healthy specimen. I rarely had to go to the doctor, though if I got a cold that affected my chest I might have a nasty cough for several weeks.

After leaving home, I discovered the delights of vegetables and later on wholemeal bread. After a year or so I noticed that my periods were no longer painful, though I didn't associate it with my improved diet. Needless to say, the constipation also improved a great deal.

Much later, after beginning to study nutrition, I started to take many dietary supplements, mainly for experimental reasons. The most welcome effect was that I began to sleep properly for the first time in my life, and had no more difficulty in falling asleep. I also no longer caught colds. If I felt one beginning I could nip it in the bud in a few hours with large doses of vitamin C powder. A quite unexpected effect of taking supplements was that my weight increased on the scales by half a stone, but my clothes size stayed exactly the same. To this day I have not been able to explain it. Possibly my bone density had improved. I certainly felt fitter, my skin improved, and I have never had any more heart pains since then.

I also experimented with diagnostic diets for food allergy and discovered that I was allergic to eggs. I didn't always get a headache when I ate them, but if I was under the slightest stress, even something as minor as not having had enough sleep, then eating even a trace of egg, as in cake or mayonnaise, would bring on a severe, all-day headache. (Without the eggs, stress alone did not cause headaches.) Avoiding eggs as well as artificial food additives improved my wind and bloating enormously. I was clearly sensitive to these substances, which were irritating my intestines. I subsequently noticed that whenever I ate foods containing sulphur dioxide preservative (such as dried fruit) I would quickly bloat up quite uncomfortably.

So for me, nutritional therapy brought benefits which I really was not expecting. I was suffering from both nutritional deficiencies and food allergies and was not aware of it. Whilst it is a common belief that all allergic reactions occur quickly and immediately on exposure to the offending substance, in reality it is all too common to have delayed or chronic reactions, or only to develop symptoms occasionally. A lot of people have allergy-related illness yet they have never associated their symptoms with any particular food.

Likewise an enormous number of people eat a good diet and it has never occurred to them that their symptoms may be due to nutritional deficiencies. But deficiency symptoms can and do exist in the presence of a good diet, since there is another very important cause of deficiency besides poor diet, and that is poor assimilation. If your digestion is not strong and healthy you can develop nutritional deficiencies just as if you were eating a very poor diet.

Nutritional therapists help food assimilation by using techniques to improve the digestion, and by treating food allergies which cause inflammation in the intestines, preventing them from absorbing food properly.

Nutritional therapy helped my symptoms by helping my body to function better. Our body contains thousands of tiny factories whose job is to manufacture the substances we need to keep us feeling well: enzymes, hormones, prostaglandins, blood corpuscles, energy, antibodies to name just a few. It is the efficiency with which it carries out these tasks which determines how well we feel and also how well we resist and fight disease. So any therapy which encourages good function can

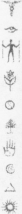

help in the fight against disease. Nutritional therapy helps by removing stressors, providing raw materials and aiding food assimilation. The presence of stressors and nutritional deficiencies can profoundly affect the functioning of the immune system, endocrine (hormonal) system, brain and nervous system, and the liver.

DO YOU NEED NUTRITIONAL THERAPY?

SOME PROBLEMS AND SYMPTOMS WHICH CAN BE DUE TO NUTRITIONAL DEFICIENCY:

Adult-onset diabetes

Birth defects

Depression

Frequent infections (eg colds, flu, thrush)

Hyperactivity in children and increasing difficulty in controlling aggression in adults

Infertility

Lack of energy

Menstrual, premenstrual and menopausal symptoms

Mental illness (some forms of)

Mood swings and other behavioural problems that seem unrelated to external events

Nausea and vomiting of pregnancy

Skin problems of all types

SOME PROBLEMS AND SYMPTOMS WHICH CAN BE DUE TO FOOD ALLERGY:

Asthma

Colitis

Eczema and psoriasis

Fluid retention and bloating

Hay fever

Hyperactivity or other behavioural disturbances in children and adults

Indigestion

Irritable bowel syndrome

Joint pains

Migraine

Severe constipation (when no other cause is found)

Sinusitis

SOME PROBLEMS AND SYMPTOMS WHICH HAVE BEEN LINKED WITH TOXIC OVERLOAD:

Asthma

Autoimmune diseases such as rheumatoid arthritis and systemic lupus erythematosus

Chronic headaches

Degenerative diseases (eg multiple sclerosis, cancers, motor neurone disease, Alzheimer's disease, Parkinsonism, osteoarthritis)

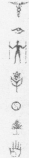

Multiple allergies and sensitivity to chemicals

Myalgic encephalomyelitis (M.E.) and chronic fatigue

Psoriasis

RESEARCH STUDY

Of 300 patients with different health problems referred for nutritional therapy by a GP in a 1993 study, the following percentages reported a 'definite, lasting improvement', usually within two months:

Headaches or migraine	85%
Digestive problems	82%
Hormone-related problems	70%
Chronic tiredness	55%
Skin diseases	54%

NUTRITIONAL DEFICIENCIES

O rthodox nutritionists and doctors maintain that nutritional deficiencies are very rare in the Western world, although they acknowledge that certain groups of people may be at risk: expectant mothers, dieters, the elderly and children. Also, most would not disagree that vegetarians who are ignorant about healthy eating are also a risk group. For instance some will simply eat chips instead of hamburger and chips, and do not know that meat should be replaced with pulses and other sources of vegetable protein.

Nutritional therapists disagree that deficiencies are rare. In our opinion they are extremely common. Our basis for this statement is that people who consult us often lose their health problems as a result of our treatments. Since our treatments usually involve either asking the client to eat more nutrient-rich foods or, if they already eat a good diet, improving food assimilation and recommending dietary supplements, we believe it is reasonable to consider that the original health problems were partially or wholly due to nutritional deficiency states.

Today this would be considered an unusual and 'unscientific' method of diagnosing nutritional deficiencies. If so, science certainly seems to have taken a step backwards. As Dr Abram

Hoffer points out, in the 1940s after it was shown that vitamin B₃ could cure pellagra, this became a diagnostic test. If the patients responded to the vitamin they received a diagnosis of pellagra. If not they were labelled with schizophrenia.

Nowadays scientists seek what they call *hard* evidence. For instance a research study measuring the blood nutrient levels of 100 people with the same symptoms, and demonstrating that they are abnormally low.

But here we get stuck on the definition of 'abnormal'. The blood is subject to what is known as 'homoeostatic control', that is to say blood nutrient levels are always more or less constant. They have to be kept constant because excessive variations could be dangerous. For instance if blood calcium levels are getting low, the body could develop a dangerous condition known as 'tetany', leading to convulsions. So the blood borrows calcium from the bones, hoping to put it back later. If the calcium shortage continues, more and more calcium will be 'borrowed' from the bones. The blood will continue to show normal calcium readings, but the bones will become demineralised and osteoporotic.

The same applies to most nutrients, and organs or structures other than the bones may be involved. As Adelle Davis, a nutritionist writing in the 1960s remarked:

'The first stage of a dietary deficiency occurs when there is failure of supply – either because food is mishandled, the diet is poorly selected, or the individual, for one of many reasons. . . has increased his needs. Failure of supply may also be initiated or aggravated by difficulties in the digestion, the absorption, or transport of nutrients within the body. Other difficulties may be created by a breakdown in enzyme systems.

'Once supply has failed for any of these reasons, there will be a drop in the blood levels of the nutrient. The blood now draws upon the tissues and when that process comes to an end, it borrows from the organ reserves. Note: Although you are well on your way towards trouble at this point, the blood levels of nutrients reveal nothing abnormal, because of the borrowing the body initiates to achieve more equitable distribution of an inadequate supply.

'Then functional disability begins – indigestion, nervousness, irritability, a tendency to weep without provocation, a shortening of the memory and attention spans, difficulty in concentration, insomnia, and bad dreams – for which the doctor's X ray, blood tests, urine analysis, stethoscope and blood-pressure instruments will find no physical justification. . .'(Adelle Davis, *Eating Right for You*, 1967).

Only if tissue and organ reserves become so depleted that the deficiency begins to show up in the blood, will a condition such as 'scurvy' or 'beri-beri' be diagnosed. About 30 people a year in Britain die from these diseases, according to a 1991 government survey.

Meanwhile, in people who never reach this drastic endpoint because their deficiency is not absolute, what damage is occurring to their ability to make hormones, corpuscles, enzymes and other substances needed for good health? Drained of the raw materials they need to make these substances, how can the organs function efficiently?

Organ biopsies (small samples of tissue) would show a deficiency state more clearly than a blood sample, but would be extremely impractical.

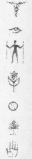

PROOF?

Shall we ever be able to convince decision-makers that nutritional deficiency is common? Is there any point in trying to do so as long as accepted criteria are so incompatible with ours? Ordinary people don't require the same sort of proof as scientists. Seeing examples of other people with similar health problems who got well after seeing a nutritional therapist may be enough proof for someone who has a lot to lose if they cannot regain their health. The fact that a lack of scientifically acceptable proof of efficacy could mean that complementary medicine might not work for them is accepted just as they accept the failure of orthodox medicine (despite its scientifically correct trials) to help them. If orthodox medicine had worked for them, they would not have needed to seek alternatives.

Until scientific criteria change, we have to go on helping people as best we can under the banner of alternative or complementary medicine. Some private laboratories are developing alternative tests for low nutrient levels, such as measuring the amount of zinc excreted in sweat, or the amount of magnesium in red blood cells. But mainstream medicine is very reluctant to accept the need for such tests or the view that problems like premenstrual syndrome or eczema can be symptoms of deficiency disease. They already have palliative drug treatments for premenstrual syndrome and eczema and see no reason to change these treatments.

We should not blame doctors for this attitude. It is a brave step for anyone in the medical profession to depart from accepted beliefs and treatment methods since staying within medical consensus (doing the same as any of their colleagues would do in a given situation) protects doctors from malpractice lawsuits.

WHAT CAUSES
NUTRITIONAL DEFICIENCIES?

There are still parts of the world where nutritional deficiency is a serious problem due to starvation and malnutrition. As a child in the 1960s I was brought up in Nigeria, and everywhere in the rural villages were children with matchstick arms and legs and the enormous pot-bellies of protein-energy malnutrition.

Our nutritional deficiency states in the industrialized world seem negligible by comparison. It is little wonder that orthodox workers, whose training in deficiency states mainly centres on the problems of the Third World, tend to be dismissive of the suggestion that nutritional deficiency is common in developed countries where we are surrounded by plenty.

The problem here is that it is not usually a lack of food which leads to deficiency states but poor nutrition education. When I worked as a nutritional therapist in a GP practice in London, I came across large numbers of people who had absolutely no idea of their body's nutritional needs. One woman existed on white flour crackers dipped in tea, and a canteen meal once a week. Another, while pregnant, ate only cheesecake and junk cereals. These people were not so short of money that they couldn't afford good food. They were lacking in education. They didn't *know* how to eat to keep healthy. It is to my mind almost criminally negligent for a school not to teach its pupils about healthy eating from the earliest age, yet, in the UK at least, nutrition and home economics is playing a smaller and smaller part in the national curriculum.

Although I was fortunate enough to work in a GP practice, most nutritional therapists in Britain are not, and must work privately. Because of this they tend to see a completely different type of client or patient. Those who pay to consult a nutritional therapist are generally very interested in food and nutrition. They have already worked at their own health, eating the healthiest diet they can imagine. Some have even taken many vitamin pills. They have decided to consult a professional nutritional therapist because they have an innate belief that food holds the key to getting well again and perhaps someone else can help them find that key.

Over and over again in these cases we come across people who have eaten an excellent diet for years, yet clearly have nutritional deficiency symptoms like premenstrual syndrome, fatigue and skin disorders. There is one school of opinion which maintains that this is because modern food is depleted by intensive farming methods. For instance although crops grown on a zinc-rich soil will pick up zinc and pass it on to us for nourishment, fertilizer products, which are intended to enrich soil that has been depleted by too many harvests, generally don't include zinc and other trace elements because the crops themselves don't need them in order to thrive.

Many fruits may not come to us straight from the tree but may first be put into cold storage for months, waiting for the price to rise. All this takes its toll on our food. Sperm counts of organic farmers, who grow crops without using pesticides and artificial fertilizers, have been shown to be double those of ordinary men, which suggests that our food is no longer of the same quality as it used to be before the practice of widespread artificial soil fertilization began after World War II. Also that our health is being affected.

There is certainly much to be said for this view, and it is also known that pollution increases our requirements for some nutrients, particularly the antioxidant vitamins and minerals (vitamins A, C and E and the mineral selenium). These nutrients can combine with toxins and escort them out of the body. They can also neutralize free radicals – harmful oxygen species like ozone which are produced by pollution, cigarette smoke and radioactivity among other things. In the process they are rapidly used up. For instance lower levels of vitamin C are found in the blood of smokers compared with non-smokers.

People who eat a borderline diet may be so finely balanced between adequacy and inadequacy that the ingestion of nutritionally depleted chemically-grown foods together with increased needs due to pollution tip them over into a deficiency state. However, I am personally not altogether convinced that the many nutritional deficiency symptoms which I come across in people who eat a *good* diet are due to these factors. At least not directly. And by a good diet I mean a varied intake of vegetables cooked carefully to conserve nutrients, wholemeal bread, dairy produce, fish, chicken, pulses, nuts or seeds, brown rice, a daily intake of fruit or fruit juice, and a restricted intake of fried and fatty foods, sugar, salt and alcohol.

Neither am I convinced that 'biochemical individuality' in the sense of variations in nutritional requirements due to ordinary genetic diversity, is the explanation. This may account for small variations in nutritional needs, but there is no reason why these should not be met by good food. I am personally convinced that most deficiency-related ill-health is due to a reduced ability to absorb and assimilate nutrients. This is discussed further in the next chapter.

VITAMIN DEPENDENCY

Occasionally, individuals do seem to have greatly increased needs. For instance there are some types of schizophrenics who have massively increased requirements for vitamin B_6 and zinc, without which they are not free of hallucinations and other symptoms. But this type of deficiency suggests some kind of malfunction rather than a natural variation in micronutrient

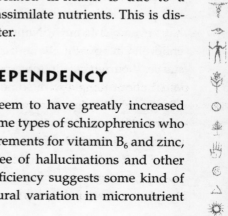

(vitamin and mineral) requirements, and is known as a vitamin 'dependency'. As to how a vitamin dependency may develop (if it is not congenital), it is certainly a fact that a period of severe nutritional deficiency may result in greatly increased requirements for individual nutrients, as happened to prisoners released from Japanese prisoner-of-war camps after World War II. A number of those with neurological symptoms were given several hundred milligrams a day of B vitamins (very large doses indeed) for what was intended to be a short period of treatment. This was effective, but the symptoms returned whenever the dosage was reduced and it took up to ten years before the neurological damage due to the deficiency had been repaired sufficiently for the veterans to be symptom-free when they stopped taking the supplements.

In the days when pellagra was common in the United States, it was observed that those who had had the disease for a long time required 600 mg of vitamin B_3 a day to keep them well. This is 50 times the dose required to prevent pellagra.

From these examples we know that historically it is certainly possible to have severe nutritional deficiency symptoms without eating a poor diet. In our modern times it is rare to develop an actual deficiency *disease*, but what about people who have had periods of relative nutritional deficiency in their lives, perhaps even before birth? National food surveys show that many children are appallingly nourished. Dieters may intermittently starve themselves for long periods to control their weight. What about people with some intestinal disorder like chronic allergy which prevents them from absorbing nutrients from their food properly? Is it not entirely possible that these people could also develop a higher than normal need for certain nutrients? Is it not also possible that the reason why nutritional therapy, with its use of dietary supplements, helps so many people with skin problems, mood changes, hormonal problems,

RICHARD: A CASE
OF NUTRITIONAL DEFICIENCY

Richard packed shelves in a supermarket and was 32 years old.
For eight years he had had what appeared to be a huge scab
measuring about two inches in diameter on his slightly balding
head.

Richard had consulted many doctors with this problem.
'They just dab at it with stuff and then send me away,' he said
in desperation. 'They won't tell me what it is and nothing
they've given me has ever stopped it.' His self-confidence had
been destroyed by this problem. He confessed that he couldn't
stop thinking about it and imagined that other people were
always looking at the scab. He would have liked to have a girl-
friend but believed that no one would want him with this
unsightly problem.

Richard had worked hard at his diet. He had grown up on a
diet of very ordinary food: 'meat and two veg', puddings,
chips, lots of sweet tea and coffee. He had never consumed
excessive amounts of sweets, chocolates or soft drinks, and his
saturated fat consumption was no higher than the average. In
the last year he had made efforts to eat more vegetables and salads, and had given up most fried foods as well as biscuits and
the occasional bar of chocolate. There was no improvement in
his scalp condition.

I explained that like his doctors I did not know what could
be causing his problem, but that skin conditions usually
responded quite well to two measures: correcting nutritional
deficiencies and taking measures to improve liver function.
Richard was prepared to go ahead and see what could be

achieved by following a nutritional programme designed on that basis.

I gave Richard a diet which completely excluded saturated fat, dairy produce and red meat, which contain arachidonic acid, a pro-inflammatory substance found in animal fats. Arachidonic acid can also be made within the body, but if excluded from foods eaten in the diet the overall body load will be decreased. The diet also excluded tea and coffee, artificial food additives and alcohol.

The nutritional deficiencies most often linked with skin problems are zinc, vitamin A and the fatty acids GLA (found in evening primrose oil) and EPA (found in fish oils). I gave Richard supplements of all these nutrients, together with a basic multivitamin and multimineral product to ensure a good balance, and also some herbs to help drain his gall bladder and aid liver function.

Nothing much seemed to happen for the first few weeks, then we noticed that as Richard's hair grew, the scab seemed to be gradually lifting off with it. By the tenth week it had grown out completely, and the skin underneath was normal.

Cases like this are not unusual. It seems so sad that more people are not aware of the benefits of nutritional therapy. Richard's confidence and sense of self-worth had been severely scarred by so many years of enduring this unsightly problem.

FOOD ABSORPTION AND ASSIMILATION

No matter how good the food we eat, if it is not well digested (broken down into individual molecules), absorbed into the blood and assimilated into cells and tissues, we can in time develop symptoms and signs of nutritional deficiency.

The first stage of digestion is the mouth. Food must be well chewed and mixed with saliva, which contains an enzyme (salivary amylase) that starts off the process of starch digestion. After swallowing, the food reaches the stomach, where it is mixed with pepsin and hydrochloric acid. Bacteria and parasites ingested with the food are killed by the acid, and the breakdown of the protein in food begins here.

Hydrochloric acid also plays an important part in the next stage of digestion. As the food leaves the stomach and enters the duodenum the acidity stimulates the liver and pancreas to release bicarbonate, which in turn raises the food's pH (makes it more alkaline). An alkaline environment is needed for the next stage of digestion. The liver (via the gall bladder) also releases bile salts, which help to emulsify fats, reducing the size of the fat droplets.

The alkalinity acts as a signal for the pancreas to release its digestive enzymes: amylase (for starch digestion), protease (for protein digestion) and lipase (for fat or 'lipid' digestion). With the aid of these enzymes starch is broken down into sugars, protein is broken down into amino acids, and fat is broken down into fatty acids and monoglycerides. Some enzymes required for the final stages of breakdown are secreted by the wall of the small intestine itself.

In a healthy person food is broken down into these smaller components and then absorbed through the wall of the duodenum and small intestine into the bloodstream (sugars and amino acids) or into the lymphatic system (fats). But amino acids and sugars cannot necessarily pass through unaided; they are carried across by a process known as 'active transport', an energy-dependent process involving carrier molecules which shift the nutrients through the epithelial cells which line the gut wall, into the bloodstream on the other side. The blood then carries the nutrients to the tissues, where cells take them up and assimilate them for various purposes. This uptake process is rarely automatic (simple diffusion); it can be quite complex, involving electrical signals, feedback mechanisms, and special 'receptors' (binding sites) which are like locks that only the right substances can open.

Vitamins are absorbed from food in a similar way to other nutrients. Fat-soluble vitamins (A, D, E, K) are absorbed together with the fats in which they are dissolved, in the lower part of the small intestine (the ileum). Any defect in fat digestion and absorption would therefore be likely to result in deficiencies of the fat-soluble vitamins.

Most of the remaining (water-soluble) vitamins are absorbed from the upper part of the small intestine (the jejunum). They diffuse through the gut wall or are actively transported across, except for vitamin B_{12}, a very large molecule which must first be combined with a protein called 'intrinsic factor' secreted by the stomach.

Some forms of minerals require an acid environment for absorption, so may only be absorbed from the duodenum, where acidity still remains after passage through the stomach. (Some mineral absorption also occurs from the colon.) Gastric acid frees trace elements such as zinc from the food complexes in which they occur. The elements can then form complexes or 'chelates' with amino acids or other substances in the gut. In this form they can be readily transported across the gut wall.

The natural absorption rate of many nutrients (including beta carotene, calcium, magnesium, and trace elements) through the gut wall can vary considerably. If the body is short of calcium, for instance, then it will allow more calcium to pass through. If a meal contains very large amounts of calcium, then most of the calcium will pass down the intestine unabsorbed. Since calcium and magnesium compete for absorption, a very calcium-rich diet could result in a considerably reduced magnesium uptake from food. There are many pairs of minerals and trace elements which 'antagonize' each other in this way. It is a reason to be cautious of taking dietary supplements for too long without professional supervision.

HYPOCHLORHYDRIA

Clearly there are opportunities for any of these processes to go wrong. Malfunctions of any of the organs described: stomach, pancreas, liver, gall bladder, gut wall, can result in impaired digestion and absorption. For example if the stomach is not acid enough, (a condition known as hypochlorhydria) the remaining processes of digestion may not be adequately triggered. Bacteria and parasites may not be killed, and may have the opportunity to infect the small intestine. Minerals may not be properly absorbed.

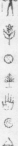

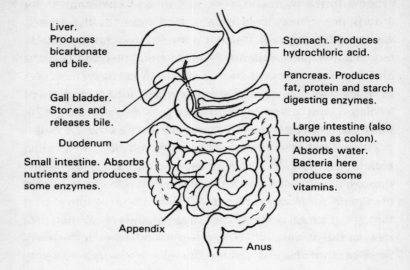

Liver. Produces bicarbonate and bile.

Stomach. Produces hydrochloric acid.

Pancreas. Produces fat, protein and starch digesting enzymes.

Gall bladder. Stores and releases bile.

Duodenum

Large intestine (also known as colon). Absorbs water. Bacteria here produce some vitamins.

Small intestine. Absorbs nutrients and produces some enzymes.

Appendix

Anus

Cross-section of small intestine (gut) wall

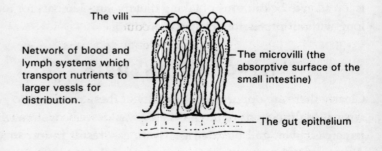

The villi

Network of blood and lymph systems which transport nutrients to larger vessls for distribution.

The microvilli (the absorptive surface of the small intestine)

The gut epithelium

The Digestive System

Some research studies suggest that up to 40 per cent of the elderly population may suffer from hypochlorhydria. So it is hardly surprising that fragile bones and osteoporosis, which suggest mineral deficiencies, are endemic among the elderly. Unfortunately standard medical procedure does not involve measuring gastric acidity and taking corrective measures. Some doctors may even give calcium carbonate supplements to these patients, not knowing that calcium and magnesium carbonate cannot be absorbed properly by hypochlorhydria sufferers.

The small intestine and sometimes the stomach can become overgrown with undesirable bacteria. This is known as dysbiosis and is thought to be quite common in cases of hypochlorhydria. Constant belching and burping can be a sign of this as the bacteria ferment the stomach contents, releasing copious quantities of carbon dioxide gas. Sometimes hydrochloric acid *is* produced but is delayed, arriving in the stomach after the food has departed, and causing burning sensations because there is nothing to buffer it.

Drugs to suppress gastric acid production are the standard orthodox treatment in these cases even though these drugs can obviously worsen hypochlorhydria.

ROSEMARY: A CASE OF HYPOCHLORHYDRIA

Rosemary had been to just about every doctor she had heard of, both orthodox and complementary. She felt desperately tired all the time. What seemed to drain her of energy most of all was the discomfort in her tummy area which would last for hours after eating. She felt as if her food would not digest. It just lay 'like a stone'. The problem had first started after a dose of antibiotics which it turned out she was allergic to and nearly died. Upon recovery her digestion was never the same again.

Rosemary's GP had given her a number of tests and con-

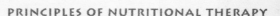

cluded that she had 'extremely high gastric acid levels'. Rosemary didn't feel that the tablets he prescribed did her much good, so she sought help elsewhere.

Another doctor diagnosed candidiasis (infestation of the small intestine with the yeast Candida albicans) and prescribed large doses of the drug nystatin. These didn't help either.

By the time Rosemary ended up with me, she was despairing of ever finding the answer to her problems, but she was slowly getting worse and didn't want to have to give up work. So she kept on trying.

Rosemary had only ever had antibiotics once in her life, so I didn't think her problem was caused by candidiasis. Candida albicans usually only thrives when the individual has taken quite a lot of antibiotics, since these kill off the friendly bacteria in the intestine which keep Candida under control.

As soon as someone tells me that food 'seems to lie like a stone' although the doctor can't find anything to account for it, I always suspect hypochlorhydria. And in Rosemary's case, where the medical tests had actually found very high levels of acid, this had to be a case of delayed acid production rather than an inability to make acid.

I decided to risk giving Rosemary hydrochloric acid supplements despite the high acidity levels which her doctor had found, and asked Rosemary to phone me instantly if any burning sensations occurred. The reason for the supplements, which were to be taken with meals, was to ensure that hydrochloric acid was in the stomach at the right time, and would therefore trigger the rest of the digestive process. Because exogenous (external) acid was provided at the right time, the reflex action which can produce excessive acid after initial hypochlorhydria, should be prevented.

I also prescribed comfrey tea. Comfrey is a particularly soothing herb for the digestive system and helps to regenerate damaged tissue. Rosemary found this treatment to be an unqualified success, particularly the comfrey tea. She had experienced no burning sensations from the hydrochloric acid supplements, and her digestion was beginning to work again. She was still tired, but it was likely that nutritional deficiencies had built up over the years that she had been ill, and the damage from these would take a little while to repair. Once these repairs could take place Rosemary would no longer need to take hydrochloric acid supplements. Her own functions would improve.

The production of adequate gastric acid and also pancreatic enzymes is dependent on an adequate intake and digestion of protein as well as zinc and other micronutrients involved in building protein-based substances: vitamin B_6, folic acid, iron and vitamin B_{12}. Long-term shortages of these nutrients and their co-factors, even if minor, can lead to shortages of enzymes and therefore to impaired protein digestion. Poor digestion is a vicious circle; it can only get poorer as less nutrients are absorbed. It can also cause chronic irritation of the intestines, damaging their ability to absorb nutrients. Improperly digested food has an irritant effect as well as providing a source of nourishment for undesirable bacteria, which produce toxic substances that may also act as irritants.

DYSBIOSIS

Dysbiosis, the overgrowth of the intestines with undesirable bacteria, is not only encouraged by hypochlorhydria but also by antibiotics, which readily destroy the friendly resident bacteria in the intestines, so allowing undesirable bacteria, which are more resistant to antibiotics, to flourish. The irritation caused by toxic substances produced by the bacteria may result in inflammation of the gut wall, which involves waterlogging of cells, and is sometimes noticeable as swelling or bloating of the abdomen. It is likely that waterlogging affects the absorptive capacity of epithelial cells and the function of carrier molecules, but the extent of malabsorption that it may cause is unknown.

Another important cause of intestinal irritation, inflammation, and waterlogging is food allergy or intolerance. Food allergy sufferers often seem to have symptoms of micronutrient (vitamin and mineral) deficiency.

Long-term irritation of the intestines, whatever the mechanisms involved, is thought to have a harmful effect not only on the intestines' ability to absorb nutrients, but also on the ability of the gut wall to prevent inadequately digested molecules from coming into contact with the bloodstream. If the integrity of the gut wall becomes impaired, allowing partially digested particles and toxic substances into the bloodstream, 'autointoxication', or the overloading of the liver with excessive detoxification work, may occur. This is thought to play a part in a number of chronic health problems, particularly fatigue and multiple allergies (see chapter on toxic overload). A loss of gut integrity is known as excessive gut permeability, or 'leaky gut syndrome'. Tests are now available for the diagnosis of a leaky gut, but nutritional therapists often diagnose it from symptom analysis alone. Food intolerance and chemical sensitivity, together with bloating, flatulence and a history of other digestive difficulties are strongly suggestive of this problem.

I would urge readers at this point to remember that we are not talking here about a proposed cause of all chronic fatigue and multiple allergy. There is no single cause. We are talking about using our knowledge of physiology and biochemistry to explore how we can work with individuals whose orthodox health carers have little to offer them, to try to understand what has happened to make them unwell and hopefully to try to reverse that process.

Apart from dysbiosis, other factors which can damage the integrity of the gut epithelium are alcohol consumption, hot chilli peppers, and aspirin-based painkillers.

Some forms of dysbiosis can have a systemic effect on the body, causing widespread malfunction. Candida albicans is probably the best known example, and is discussed in the next chapter.

The two most obvious signs that food is not being properly digested (whatever the cause) are the presence of much undigested food in the stools, and persistent intestinal wind or flatulence. Much flatulence can occur when undigested food is seized and consumed by bacteria, which ferment it, producing gas.

ASSIMILATION AND CELLULAR UPTAKE

Once nutrients enter the bloodstream, they have to be taken up by the cellular systems which use them. One of the principal problems which can occur with this process is that some toxins commonly present in the body appear to be very similar to essential nutrients. For instance the chemistry of lead resembles calcium so greatly that if calcium is in short supply and there is plenty of lead available, then lead can be absorbed instead of calcium both from the gastrointestinal tract (if ingested) and from the bloodstream into cellular systems.

The problem is that lead cannot perform the same tasks as calcium, so it disrupts the function of the cellular systems which are attempting to use it, and these effectively become calcium-deficient. Also, as described by Professor Derek Bryce-Smith in 1983, lead interferes with the synthesis of neurotransmitters (essential messenger substances used by the brain and nervous system) and can produce a false neurotransmitter

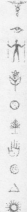

called ALA, which competes with the real neurotransmitter GABA. GABA is needed to prevent the nervous system from becoming overactive. An individual whose GABA receptors are instead picking up ALA may develop a lack of inhibitory control. It is not difficult to see why high lead levels in the body are linked with hyperactivity and learning difficulties in children and aggressive or sociopathic behaviour in adults.

Countless other toxins can have similar disruptive effects on metabolism and function. They need not be present in large quantities to have these effects.

It is also possible that the mechanisms which pump specific nutrients from the blood into the cells can become damaged by toxins, or even by viruses or other micro-organisms. Symptoms may then occur which suggest that these nutrients are deficient even when large amounts of them are present in the bloodstream. In the illness known as ME (myalgic encephalomyelitis) or chronic fatigue syndrome, for example, sufferers have muscle pain thought to be due to chronic muscular spasm, a common symptom of magnesium deficiency. Magnesium supplementation appears to make little difference to sufferers in the short term, but magnesium injections, which flood the cell with very large amounts of magnesium, appear to offer temporary relief. It is thought that in these cases some damage may have occurred to magnesium uptake mechanisms, perhaps by unknown toxins.

When deficiency symptoms seem to occur in the absence of any dietary inadequacy, this is known as a 'functional' deficiency. The nutritional therapist will attempt to improve the absorption and assimilation of the nutrient(s) in question. This may involve working to eliminate any toxic substances which may be helping to impair the use of the nutrient(s) in question.

6

CANDIDIASIS

C andida albicans is a common yeast found in most people. Under normal circumstances it causes no problems, but it can multiply in the mouth, vagina or intestines, forming a white overgrowth known as thrush. Thrush in the intestines – usually called candidiasis – is a form of dysbiosis. It is particularly encouraged if antibiotics have been taken, since they kill the natural bacterial population of the intestines which normally keep the yeast under control. Yeasts themselves are not affected by antibiotics. Other factors which encourage candidiasis are a weakened immune system (after a debilitating illness, for example), oral contraceptives, steroid drugs, tobacco smoking and sugar consumption. As we know, yeasts thrive on sugar.

The Candida yeast cells are thought to have fungus-like properties and to attach themselves to the intestine by means of 'roots'. These roots may damage the wall of the intestine, making it more permeable and causing the 'leaky gut' referred to in the previous chapter. Tiny particles of partially digested foods can escape into the bloodstream. The immune system may attack these particles as it can't distinguish between undigested food and bacteria. The resulting immune reaction causes inflammation, often leading to symptoms like bloating and diarrhoea. But the inflammation need not be confined to the gut; inflammation frequently occurs in other parts of the body such as the head (migraine) or the skin (rashes). These are thought of as allergic symptoms. Strictly speaking they are symptoms of food intolerance and not classical allergies. If the foods did not 'leak' into the bloodstream in a partially digested state, the reactions would probably not occur.

As discussed in the previous chapter, poor digestion and absorption of food can occur when the intestines are inflamed, which in turn may lead to nutritional deficiencies and so to further weakening of the immune system. Apart from causing poor food assimilation due to inflamed intestines, a thick coating of Candida on the inside of the intestines can partially block the absorption of nutrients from the diet. Some of the symptoms often associated with Candida infestation, such as increased tiredness, skin problems, PMS and period pains, nervous problems and hormonal imbalances, are probably partly due to acquired nutritional deficiencies.

Fatigue is probably the most common problem associated with candidiasis. The yeast produces toxic waste products, which further stress the immune system and liver and can leave the sufferer with severe fatigue and a feeling of being drained. Muscular weakness and/or pain is also common. The best known of these toxins is acetaldehyde, which is the same chemical that is found in excessive amounts in cheap wine and is responsible for hangovers. This is not surprising since Candida is a yeast and ferments food into alcohol and associated by-products. Many Candida sufferers report feeling as if they are chronically hung over. For reasons probably to do with the development of chemical sensitivities as a result of a toxic overload on the liver, the sufferer may also feel very unwell in the presence of strong perfumes, fumes and other inhalant factors.

Candidiasis is often associated with poor blood sugar balance which can make sufferers feel depressed, with emotions difficult to control, irritability, poor concentration or drowsiness. The yeast does appear to be capable of profoundly affecting the hormonal (endocrine) system in general. Candida albicans is thought to be able to migrate from the gut to other parts of the body, and the effects of this are as yet poorly understood. Biologist and natural medicine practitioner Sherridan Stock says:

> Candida and its toxins appear to exert a direct cytotoxic effect on the adrenal glands via free radical activity. Another mechanism suggested by our testing is that of Candida-induced autoimmune damage. Several studies do, in fact, implicate Candida as a major cause of autoimmunity since it can reduce suppressor T-cell activity. We wonder whether the presence of Candida and its toxins within a tissue causes the body to regard that tissue as nonself and therefore to initiate autoimmune attack.

[Autoimmune damage is caused by the immune system failing to distinguish between self and non-self, and starting to attack the body's own cells. The suppressor T-cells are white blood cells which normally help to prevent such an over-reaction of the immune system.]

There is also evidence, says Sherridan Stock, that Candida albicans possesses receptor sites which can bind adrenal hormones, thyroid hormones and other hormones, and render them unavailable to the body, thus causing severe disruption to metabolism and function.

The Candida yeast is present in everyone's intestines in small amounts. Since there is no widely available test which definitively proves that an individual has *excessive* amounts of this yeast, most doctors will not consider it seriously as a cause of chronic fatigue or other common symptoms. Although it is slowly becoming acknowledged that fungal infestation is becoming a more widespread phenomenon, orthodox workers still believe that it only occurs systemically in life-threatening illnesses such as cancer and Aids.

The anti-fungal drug nystatin is commonly prescribed by doctors for vaginal thrush. It can also be taken internally, and some doctors will prescribe it. To be effective it needs to be taken as a powder in fairly large amounts, and, being poorly absorbed, it will only act on the gastrointestinal tract. Another widely prescribed anti-fungal drug is amphotericin but this is severely hepatotoxic (damaging to the liver).

Occasionally patients react severely to nystatin. Also, many appear to find that their Candida returns as soon as they stop taking it. One explanation could be the 'lawn-mower' effect – that is that nystatin can kill off the top layer of Candida in the intestine, but not the roots, thus allowing Candida to grow again. Another could be that the doctor may not give proper nutritional counselling for Candida control, may not take important preventive action such as taking women off the contraceptive pill, and so on.

For nutritional therapists and other practitioners, there has been confusion for some years over diagnosing and treating candidiasis, and the diagnosis has become a kind of 'bandwagon', over-used because it has been heavily popularized. In fact all the symptoms of candidiasis are non-specific, and can also be symptoms of allergy, nutritional deficiency and/or poisoning by toxins from sources other than Candida albicans (for instance other micro-organisms, or chemical agents).

The experienced nutritional therapist will look for a history of recent or repeated past use of antibiotics as the main diagnostic criterion for candidiasis, since such a history practically guarantees the presence of significant quantities of the Candida yeast. Whether or not this presence is responsible for all the patient's current symptoms is another matter, and may have to be determined at a later stage by assessing the outcome of prescribing an anti-Candida regime.

A CASE OF CANDIDIASIS

Barbara had had asthma since birth. It was quite severe, and her life was threatened on more than one occasion. She was taking two drugs for the prevention of asthma attacks, and also had a Ventolin inhaler to stop an attack should one occur. She used the inhaler daily. The attacks did not seem to be precipitated by anything in particular. Barbara had also suffered from regular chest infections all her life, and had taken an incredible quantity of antibiotics.

Asthma can be a very serious disease. Although it is occasionally due to a single food allergy such as dairy produce, and sufferers may lose their symptoms completely after beginning a diet which avoids the offending food, in some sufferers it is an extremely complex condition with a multifactorial aetiology, that is to say many factors operating together can be involved in its development.

Nutritional therapists always approach asthma by starting with a hypoallergenic diet – a diet which avoids the most common food allergens and also removes a number of nutritional stressors from the diet (see more about this in Chapter 11). I also gave Barbara counselling on the house dust mite, which most asthma sufferers are known to be allergic to. Oddly enough, her doctor had never done this. Barbara began to keep her bed and bedroom a strictly no-mite area, and to keep her bedroom window open at night. These measures and the diet together resulted in a 50 per cent reduction in asthma attacks. Barbara appeared to be sensitive to a number of foods, including wheat, dairy produce, artificial colourings in food, alcohol, yeast, citrus fruit and fish.

For the time being we kept Barbara on a diet of chicken, rice and vegetables to stabilize her as much as possible. The second most obvious priority was to begin detoxifying her body, since the presence of multiple allergies strongly suggests a toxic overload, and this was also likely to account for her residual asthma symptoms.

Barbara's long history of antibiotic use suggested that her intestines might contain a good deal of Candida albicans, which would certainly encourage a toxic overload, so we started her on a natural anti-fungal regime. She was already on a diet free of added sugar, on which the Candida yeast would normally thrive. I ensured that she consumed oils only in the form of cold-pressed olive oil, which has a mildly anti-fungal action, and asked her to eat garlic, onions and leeks regularly, which have a similar effect although unfortunately once cooked garlic loses most of its anti-fungal properties.

Before and during treatment with specific anti-fungal agents, it is advisable to give liver herbs, which help to drain the liver and gall bladder. This helps to prevent the Candida 'die-off' reaction, a reaction involving severe malaise which can occur when Candida albicans dies and releases large quantities of toxins. These toxins are absorbed into the blood and have to be processed by the liver and their remains stored in the gall bladder for excretion via the intestines. For this reason it is vitally important to keep the patient's bowels moving regularly.

A number of harmless, natural anti-fungal agents are now available to nutritional therapists, for example Acidophilus supplements, caprylic acid and allicin extracted from raw garlic. Shortly after Barbara began her anti-Candida regime, she started to perceive a fungus-like taste constantly at the back of her throat. This was unrelated to the taste of the products she was using, and was clearly the result of Candida albicans destruction and breakdown.

Barbara had not had a cold since beginning her treatment with me, but at this point an infection did develop, and was probably encouraged by the stress her body was undergoing from Candida die-off. However, it did not develop into her chest as it had always done in the past, and it did in fact assist her treatment. The cold caused Barbara to expectorate enormous quantities of creamy white mucus, something which had never happened to her before. We assumed that the white colour was due to her lungs releasing some of the Ventolin powder which must have accumulated in them over the years. Barbara felt very much better after her cold.

After six months' treatment, Barbara's asthma attacks were down to about one per month, a result that she was very pleased with. There was every chance that after a few more years' work on her health, Barbara's body would be strong enough to resist asthma completely.

7

ALLERGY

If we are allergic to strawberries or shellfish, we know about it, because we come up in a rash or get a headache, for instance, whenever we eat them. Most people do not eat these foods very often, and the allergic reaction can be clearly linked with the food once it has happened a few times.

On the other hand if we are allergic or 'sensitive' to something we eat or drink every day – such as milk, wheat, sugar, yeast, egg or food additives – we may not associate our symptoms with these foods. Regular exposure to an allergen forces the body to try to adapt to it – for example by increasing the output of adrenal hormones to suppress an inflammatory reaction. When symptoms occur they are usually either chronic (such as fatigue or eczema), intermittent with no seeming pattern (such as migraine or headaches) or only occur when the sufferer is tired or under stress – perhaps because the adrenal coping mechanism has been overloaded.

It is important to remember that the allergic symptoms can be perpetuated even if the amounts of allergen eaten or drunk are very small indeed, provided that consumption is regular enough.

Some of us are born allergic. These individuals are known as *atopic*, and their allergies as *atopic allergies*. This is uncontroversial, and doctors are happy to diagnose such people as allergic to house dust mite, animal fur, pollen and so on. However, most doctors' criteria for allergy diagnosis require that the reaction should be fairly rapid and easy to associate with the problem substance (for example if a weal appears in skin prick testing with a small amount of the offending substance). The type of food allergy which involves delayed, chronic or intermittent symptoms is not considered to be 'true' allergy, and it is common practice for doctors to accuse such patients of inventing their symptoms for psychiatric reasons.

Many people develop food sensitivities later in life. They do not usually suspect that they have become allergic to something they have eaten all their lives, and neither do most doctors. Symptoms like diarrhoea, fatigue, migraine and fluid retention are usually investigated only with a view to determining whether a disease may be present, and if none is found, the patient is pronounced well and healthy and given palliative medication like anti-diarrhoeal products, tranquillizers and painkillers which may have to be taken for life.

It is not known exactly how an allergy develops, but we can make some calculated guesses.

Firstly the sufferer may have had the allergy since a much earlier age without realizing it because the adrenal coping mechanisms (for instance natural cortisone production) were masking the symptoms.

Secondly, people with leaky gut syndrome are likely to experience some kind of reaction after eating foods which are not completely digested. Undigested or partially digested food particles are not designed to come into contact with the bloodstream, but in someone with a leaky gut they do, and may act as antigens (that is to say may provoke an immune reaction).

It should be remembered that a leaky gut does not necessarily 'leak' undigested food all the time. There may be times

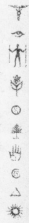

when it is less permeable, in which case the foods which usually provoke symptoms may be eaten without causing problems. This is one of the reasons why allergy diagnosis is so problematic. Conventional doctors expect allergic symptoms to be repeatable on demand.

An overload of the body's detoxification systems is also likely to lead to food-related symptoms. Foods contain many natural chemicals which are mildly toxic but which in a healthy person are easily neutralized by the liver. These are sometimes known as secondary plant metabolites. If the liver's detoxification enzymes are, on certain days, inadequate to deal with these toxins, the individual may develop symptoms after eating a particular food or food family which contains the toxins. These are not in fact symptoms of allergy but symptoms of mild poisoning. There is every reason why sensitive cells such as those in the brain, spinal cord and immune system might begin to act abnormally under such circumstances. The larger the quantities of a particular food or food family that are consumed, the worse the symptoms are likely to be. An example of such a food family might be the deadly nightshade family, which includes potatoes, tomatoes, peppers, aubergine and tobacco. All these plants are a source of alkaloids which would be extremely toxic if consumed in large amounts.

Detoxification pathways can become overloaded or dysfunctional in two ways: from excessive exposure to toxins, and from an inadequate supply of nutrients needed for the detoxification process (eg molybdenum, vitamin C, beta carotene, glutathione and other antioxidants).

ALLERGY TESTING

There are several methods of testing for allergies or sensitivities. Skin prick tests and patch tests are commonly used by doctors, and are good for substances which come into contact with the skin or nasal passages. Blood tests are also available, which use a number of different methods to determine whether blood cells show changes when exposed to foods being tested. These changes are thought to indicate that the food is allergenic to that individual. However blood tests are thought to be at best about 70 per cent accurate and indeed this is not surprising since foods would not normally come into contact with the blood in a healthy individual but should first be digested into their molecular components.

Applied kinesiology, vega testing and dowsing are used by some complementary medicine practitioners in testing for allergies. Kinesiology involves testing the strength of muscles. If a particular muscle weakens when the body is exposed to a particular food, this is thought to indicate an allergy to that food. Vega testing measures the electrical resistance of the skin, and again is thought to be able to detect allergies by abnormal readings on exposure to different foods. Dowsing involves the use of a pendulum by psychically gifted individuals. The pendulum is held over a food and 'asked' whether the patient is allergic to that food. The direction in which the pendulum swings indicates 'yes' or 'no'.

In the hands of some practitioners these can be useful tools, but in the hands of others this is not always so, no matter how good their training. According to the experts these methods do seem to depend to some extent on factors such as the practitioner's unique unconscious gifts, the patient's mental attitude, or even geomagnetic forces which may be present.

Challenge testing is the method favoured by most nutritional therapists. This requires a careful protocol of prior avoidance of suspected problem foods, followed by challenges for five days at a time (or lesser periods if symptoms occur) for each food, and should be carried out under the guidance of

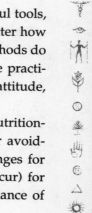

a practitioner who is aware of the potential meaning of the different outcomes of testing.

Usually only foods which the patient commonly eats every day need be tested. These will usually be wheat, dairy produce, eggs and yeast. Other foods can be identified by keeping a food and symptom diary.

Many allergy sufferers tell practitioners that they don't eat egg, or yeast, or dairy produce. In fact these foods are eaten far more commonly than most people realize. Apart from omelettes, quiches and egg sandwiches, eggs can be ingested in cakes, pasta, ready-made desserts, glazed pastry, mayonnaise, many types of vegetable or fish pâté and several different brands of ice cream. Dairy produce is present in small amounts in a lot of processed foods, which may contain small quantities of dried milk powder, whey, lactose (milk sugar) or casein (milk protein). This is one of the reasons why it is so important to carry out testing under the supervision of an experienced nutritional therapist.

Challenge testing is the only method which takes into account the fact that substantial chemical changes occur to food during the digestive process. In fact one of the keys to avoiding allergy is a strong pancreas and digestive juices, which break down food making it less allergenic. It is also important to have a healthy intestine which does not 'leak' partly digested food particles into the bloodstream, as may occur in individuals whose intestines have been damaged by Candida albicans or by a long history of inflammation in the intestines.

SEVERE MULTIPLE ALLERGIES

Occasionally a patient is so severely allergic to so many foods or environmental factors that it will be difficult to maintain a diet that is varied enough for good health. In such cases

A CASE OF MULTIPLE ALLERGY

Lorraine was a personal assistant aged 45, and consulted me because of an angry red rash which covered almost the whole left side of her face, making her look as if she had been scalded. There was another rash on her neck, which was slightly raised and purple in colour.

Lorraine had worked extremely hard to try to eradicate these rashes. She had read many health and nutrition books, taken vitamins, followed diets and avoided substances like tea and coffee, salt and sugar. She had identified a number of common foods that seemed to aggravate her skin problem, including wheat and dairy produce, red meat, eggs, citrus fruit, peppers, oats and shellfish. Avoiding such foods brought temporary relief, only to be followed by increasing sensitivity to yet another food, as her diet became more restricted. She decided to consult me because she felt that her diet was becoming dangerously limited, and she was worried that she might begin to develop nutritional deficiencies. She also seemed to be rapidly approaching the point where anything she ate would cause her skin to flare up.

Lorraine's main priority was clearly to eat a more varied diet so that she would not develop nutritional deficiencies or further allergies. In a multiple allergy sufferer, regular consumption of the same foods is likely to overload the detoxification pathways for the secondary plant metabolites found in those foods, thus seeming to result in an acquired allergy to these foods.

I asked Lorraine to write down a list of the foods which always caused a severe reaction, and those which caused only mild symptoms. There were only a few seriously problematic foods, so I asked Lorraine to continue avoiding these, but to

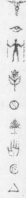

reintroduce the remaining foods back into her diet. But I did want her to minimize her exposure to these foods, in order not to overload her detoxification pathways. The answer to this was a 'rotation diet'. I asked Lorraine to cut some paper up into squares. On each square she was to write down a food that she could tolerate well, or which, when it provoked symptoms, did so only intermittently or produced only a mild reaction. Lorraine was then to divide these pieces of paper into four piles, with each pile representing one day. This resulted in about eight foods for each day. Lorraine was to swap the foods around to ensure that the foods were fairly evenly distributed according to whether they were protein, carbohydrate or fat-based, fruits, vegetables and so forth. She was then to eat each of these foods only once on the appropriate day, and after the fourth day to start all over again. The result was that she ate each food only once in a four-day period.

Skin problems of this type can be partly due to nutritional deficiencies, particularly vitamin A, zinc, and the fatty acids GLA (found in evening primrose oil) and EPA (found in fish oil). These may be primary nutritional deficiencies (due to dietary inadequacy) or functional, secondary deficiencies caused by dysfunctional metabolism. I gave Lorraine a multi-vitamin and mineral preparation, plus a little extra zinc, a combined GLA/EPA product, and some herbs to help her liver function.

At Lorraine's two-week follow-up, there was no change in her skin condition, but she reported being able to tolerate her rotation diet without bringing about any flare-ups. She was very pleased with this, although she found the diet difficult. I reassured her that it was purely a short-term diet.

At four weeks, the skin was beginning to improve slightly, and at six weeks there was a noticeable change for the better. By the eighth week the facial rash had disappeared, and only the neck rash remained. This was less angry. At this stage I allowed Lorraine to relax her diet, continuing to avoid her most problematic foods, but eating other foods without such strict regard to rotation. This did not result in any deterioration, and the improvement continued. By the twelfth week, Lorraine was sufficiently improved to be discharged from my care with a maintenance diet and a mild supplementation regime.

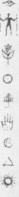

8

TOXIC OVERLOAD

I t is the detoxification system's job to deal with all foreign, abnormal or toxic substances in the body, and render them harmless. Modern pollution can be a considerable burden on the detoxification system, but it is not confined to pollution created by others. We can bring pollution into our own homes by the products and services we use. Common sources of home pollution are:

- Dry cleaning fumes

- Chemical-filled soap-powders and detergents

- Artificial air fresheners

- Strong-smelling fabric conditioners

- Household sprays

- Cosmetic aerosols and sprays, e.g. deodorants, hairspray, perfume

- Strong-smelling polishes, toilet cleaners and carpet cleaners

- Unnecessary medications or recreational drugs

- Fumes from gas cookers and central heating

- Fumes from garages built underneath bedrooms or adjacent to living quarters

- Tobacco smoke

- Mould from damp surroundings

- Dust

- Formaldehyde gas released by new carpets and furnishings

- Wood preservative

- Fly spray and other insecticides

- Artificial food additives

There are 60,000 chemicals in current commercial production. 3,000 of these are used as food additives, and 800 are found in drinking water. We can absorb pollutants from traffic fumes, factory and power station discharges into air, rivers and seas; food contaminated with pesticides, antibiotic drugs and industrial fall-out on to crops and animal feed; tap water, and even fresh country air. Wherever we live we are likely to have pesticides in our blood. They are in our food, our water, and the air we breathe. 'There is no need for concern as the amounts are so small,' say governments. Yet in Britain alone one billion gallons of pesticide a year are sprayed on to our food: one billion gallons of deadly poison.

Governments like to keep quiet about effects such as 'spray-drift' – the cloud of tiny pesticide droplets which floats away from the crop it is aimed at. Between 20 and 50 per cent of the spray can drift away and blow into neighbouring gardens and towns, to be breathed in by an unsuspecting public.

Don't imagine you are safe if you live in a city. Spraydrift from as far away as Africa can end up in Europe and America. More locally, pesticide is sprayed on pavements and parks, used in gardens, as wood preservatives, on footpaths, road margins and in buildings.

The chemicals soon soak into the water table, the underground water which ends up in our public water system. In the two years between 1985 and 1987 the limits for pesticide residues in public water were broken about 300 times in England and Wales.

The amount of pesticide which remains on our food is not great, but a 1983 UK survey revealed that just over a third of fruit and vegetables, together with foods such as bran, sausages, burgers and cheese, contained detectable residues. Apples and oranges are deliberately coated with a thin layer of pesticide-impregnated wax.

Higher levels of pesticide residue may be found in foods imported from the Third World, because farmers there are often not properly trained in their use. Ill-health due to hazardous pesticide dumps in Africa is widespread according to *Pesticide News*, the journal of the UK's Pesticides Trust. Some countries receive large 'donations' of pesticides which they have not requested and do not need. Companies do this because it may be cheaper to get rid of chemicals which have been banned in their own country than to find methods of disposing of them locally.

Whether or not we need pesticides is a complex issue. What we do know is that insects rapidly become immune to them. We also know that pesticides damage and kill our wildlife generally. But how much damage are humans suffering from pesticides?

The damage caused depends on the particular chemicals and the amount of exposure. For instance, the organochlorine insecticides (DDT-like compounds such as Lindane, Dieldrin and Aldrin) can produce tremors, twitching and convulsions, dizziness, hyperexcitability, sensitivity to noise, headaches and liver damage.

Organophosphorus insecticides (such as Malathion, Dimethoate and Dichlorvos) also damage the nervous system. In fact nerve gases for use in chemical warfare are a by-product of research into these compounds. Symptoms of acute poisoning include tremors, dizziness, convulsions, flu-like sympvomiting, lung failure and heart-block.

Thousands of people have suffered acute pesticide poisoning (symptoms or illness clearly linked with one or more incidents of pesticide exposure). But the burden of proof is always on the sufferer. Because of the technical difficulties of such proof, sufferers are rarely able to sue those responsible for their illness even though in some cases severe disability results.

Some chronic health problems such as asthma, epilepsy, repeated miscarriage or cancer are known to occur more frequently among those suffering long-term exposure to smaller amounts of pesticide, but this can never be legally proven. For instance, although a lot of pesticides are known carcinogens, many cannot be tested for in human body fluids. Even if they can be detected, it would be impossible to prove that it was one particular chemical which caused that person's illness when so many potentially cancer-causing substances are surrounding us all. Governments' attitudes are that if you have a pesticide-related problem, it is likely to be 'idiosyncratic'; in other words it's *your* fault, not the pesticides, so hard luck.

Government committees which in theory are supposed to assess whether a pesticide should or should not be allowed on the market may not even be consulted. In many cases they have been refused access to testing data. 'The 'testing method' often consists of waiting a few years to see if the product causes any problems,' says Dr Charlie Clutterbuck, an anti-pesticide campaigner in the UK. 'When it does, it's often up to campaigners to get it banned.'

Every time a pesticide is banned another one takes its place before long. We are simply not going to see less of this variety of pollution until there is more support for the organic movement. The only reason why pesticide-grown produce still exists is because people buy it. Buy organic instead and treat the extra expense as a donation to the fight against pesticides. As organic food becomes more widely produced, the price will come down.

Our body burden of toxic cocktails may gradually increase over the years since many of these substances are not readily excreted. The very high incidence of cancers now sweeping the Western world is like the death of the miner's canary. In the old days, when miners had no way of knowing whether toxic methane gas was present in a mine, they would take a canary in a cage to work with them. If the canary became ill, it was a sign to quickly vacate the mine.

At the beginning of the twentieth century, cancer was a rare disease. Now in some countries one in three people will contract it. In a recent radio programme a listener commented that every single house in the street in which he lived had a cancer sufferer.

Apart from being capable of disrupting body processes and interfering with nutrient absorption and utilization, many pollutants also damage the body by generating free (oxidizing) radicals. Free radicals are destructive types of oxygen molecules that are capable of initiating the changes responsible for causing cancer. The body itself produces some free radicals, which it uses to destroy bacteria. It then neutralizes these free radicals, making them harmless with nutrients known as antioxidants (among them vitamins A, C and E, and beta carotene) obtained from the diet. The nutrients are destroyed in the process. The body can also manufacture antioxidant enzymes to carry out a similar task, such as glutathione peroxidase, which is dependent on an adequate supply of the amino acid glutathione and the mineral selenium, now officially recognized to be dangerously deficient in the British diet and in other countries with low soil selenium levels.

Unlike the body, pollutants can generate dangerously large quantities of these free radicals. For instance benzopyrenes in diesel smoke are some of the most potent carcinogens known to man. For obvious reasons their dangers are not widely publicized, but every diesel engine which is improperly tuned and belches smoke should be reported immediately to the authorities.

Nuclear radiation, the most potent weapon of mass destruction in existence, exerts its harmful effects primarily by the creation of free radicals.

Toxins are not always man-made. Each of us consumes toxic substances every day of our lives when we eat common vegetables such as potatoes, celery, parsnips and mushrooms. Many plants contain toxins known as secondary plant metabolites. These are produced by plants for their own protection, to stop animals and insects from consuming too much of a particular species and threatening its survival. In small amounts most of these toxins do us no harm, although there have been a number of deaths as a result of solanine poisoning from potatoes, for instance.

Don't let this put you off eating vegetables. Your liver has been evolving enzymes for thousands of years to cope with secondary plant metabolites, safely detoxifying them provided your diet is varied and you do not consume too much of any one type. But should starvation strike, and only one type of plant food be available, as happened in a community in India in 1960 when there was an epidemic of poisoning by toxic lathyrogens due to an over-consumption of chick peas, you may not be so lucky!

Toxic ammonia is produced by eating meat and other protein foods. Again, a healthy liver can detoxify reasonable amounts of ammonia without problems. Endotoxins produced by the bacterial flora in the gut are another source of toxicity. Increased gut permeability ('leaky gut') can present a considerable challenge to liver detoxification because of the greatly increased uptake of gut toxins.

Clearly we live in a hostile environment whether or not we are being polluted by man-made chemicals, and only our liver stands between us and death by poisoning.

DETOXIFICATION

Researchers in the USA have found that the liver's detoxification ability in apparently healthy individuals can vary over a 60-fold range. This will not be reflected in the conventionally used liver pathology tests, which measure liver enzymes in blood. It is identified by liver function tests: challenging the liver with a substance that it has to detoxify (such as caffeine) and measuring the rate at which it does so.

In the liver, all ingested and microbe-produced toxins undergo two processes, known as Phase I and Phase II detoxification (or biotransformation). Phase I alters substances through a chemical reaction known as oxidation, using enzymes known collectively as cytochrome P-450 mixed-function oxidase enzymes. Toxins are transformed, for instance, into alcohols, then into aldehydes, and finally into acids which can be excreted via the kidneys; or sometimes the intermediate products are diverted into Phase II detoxification. Different toxins stimulate the production of different enzymes. Phase I detoxification requires the adequate presence of a number of nutrients, including magnesium, iron, molybdenum, B vitamins, zinc, vitamin C and essential fatty acids.

Aldehydes may be known to some readers as toxic chemicals found in cheap wine, commonly associated with 'hangovers'. They are also produced by the yeast Candida albicans. But aldehydes are also produced by the liver during the process of detoxifying a wide variety of chemicals. People who regularly suffer from hangover-like headaches even when they haven't consumed any alcohol may in fact be experiencing a build-up of aldehydes due to a defect in their detoxification pathways. Defects occur when an important enzyme or other substance isn't produced when needed. The next stage of biotransformation doesn't take place properly, so a kind of traffic-jam effect occurs as aldehydes and other highly toxic intermediate substances accumulate. Other toxic intermediates include epoxides and Valium-like substances (known as 'endogenous benzodiazepines') or chloral hydrate – identical to the knock-out drug more commonly known as the 'Mickey Finn'. Sometimes the intermediate substance is more toxic than the original. For instance cigarette smoke is non-toxic until it has been oxidized by the liver.

People with an excess of these intermediates don't necessarily feel hung over or sleepy or experience other adverse reactions all the time. It may take certain foods to trigger off the symptoms, which the sufferer may then identify as a 'wheat allergy', an intolerance to sugar or a tendency to feel sleepy after lunch. But these toxins do not just interfere with brain function. They can also damage cellular and enzyme function through powerful free radical activity, leading to a reduced ability to produce energy, for instance. The immune system may also be affected – not necessarily by simply becoming less resistant to infections. One particularly dangerous malfunction of the immune system is 'autoimmunity', when the immune system fails to tell the difference between the body's own cells and foreign invaders, and attacks and destroys the body itself. There is now an increasing following for the theory that autoimmunity is the most likely explanation for Aids, among other diseases. It is especially interesting that those who succumb to Aids often have a history of high exposure to xenobiotics, whether through drug abuse or regular use of antibiotics and other prescription drugs, and therefore a greater likelihood that their liver's detoxification capacity may become overwhelmed. The recent massive worldwide trial of the toxic drug AZT may have masked the possibility that the drug itself might actually contribute to the progress of Aids, because the study was so large. Few Aids sufferers and HIV+ individuals did not take part in it.

Phase II detoxification may follow on from Phase I, or chemicals may enter it straight away. Among other things it is inhibited by the food additives tartrazine (yellow colouring) and vanillin (artificial vanilla flavour found in most brands of chocolate).

Phase II involves the 'conjugation' of aldehydes and other toxins: a molecule is added to the toxin, converting it to a water-soluble form which can be excreted. The nutrients glycine, glutathione, selenium and sulphate are required for Phase II detoxification. Dietary selenium intake is known to be dangerously low in some parts of the world. In the UK the average consumption is only 34 micrograms a day, 6 micrograms below the level acknowledged to result in almost certain deficiency. The antioxidant enzyme glutathione peroxidase, which is an essential enzyme involved in the detoxification of peroxide, a dangerous free radical, is dependent on selenium, and cannot be produced without it. The body attempts to compensate for deficient production of glutathione peroxidase by producing hypochlorite ions. But in the presence of too much hypochlorite, free amino acids can turn into aldehydes; for instance the amino acid glycine becomes the dangerous toxin formaldehyde.

The body's ability to form sulphate may also be impaired. Sulphate is not normally ingested in the diet since it is inorganic. It is formed from the amino acid cysteine by a process known as sulphoxidation. Researchers at the Breakspear Hospital for Environmental Medicine in England have found that most patients with multiple chemical sensitivities (unpleasant reactions to small amounts of pollutants and other chemicals) have a sulphoxidation deficit – they cannot make enough sulphate.

Migraine sufferers who react to chocolate, cheese and oranges are particularly thought to have a problem with sulphate production. The detoxification of tyramine in cheese and octopamine in oranges (both naturally occurring substances), the contraceptive pill, hormone replacement therapy, paracetamol and other drugs, phenols present in home cleaning products etc., is dependent on the conjugation of these substances with sulphate, and will not be able to continue if sulphate runs out. This has been confirmed by researchers at Birmingham University's Department of Biochemistry in the UK, measuring the metabolism of paracetamol. These researchers have also found that sufferers from degenerative diseases of the nervous system (Parkinsonism, motor neurone disease – also known as ALS) and Alzheimer's disease, have a markedly reduced sulphoxidation capacity. They have published reports in the *Lancet* warning that these patients are likely to be more susceptible to xenobiotics.

It has always been known that poor liver detoxification can produce encephalopathy (brain damage), hallucinations and altered thinking processes, as in the chronic alcoholic with cirrhosis of the liver. These symptoms have conventionally been attributed to an excess of ammonia, which the liver has the task of detoxifying. As our understanding of liver detoxification processes improves, it becomes clear that liver dysfunction can give rise to a very broad spectrum of potential symptoms and degenerative processes, and that so far researchers have only scratched the surface of this subject.

TREATMENT

So far we have looked at some of the complexities of body processes and how they can go wrong. Orthodox nutritionists often deny that these processes frequently can and do go wrong. This is probably due to a belief that if such malfunctions are occurring then the medical system will pick up on them and apply effective orthodox solutions. For instance I have heard conventional nutritionists make statements like 'It is wrong to advertise evening primrose oil as a necessary supplement for people who cannot metabolize essential fatty acids properly. There is no need for anyone to take evening primrose oil supplements.' Such people go on to criticize doctors who prescribe dietary supplements for problems like eczema and premenstrual syndrome, arguing that 'according to clinical trials they are not effective treatments'.

An eminent textbook for orthodox nutritionists states:

[One] pharmacological agent in food that has been linked to migraine headaches is the vasoactive amine phenylethylamine, which is found in chocolate. However, this area is still controversial, since other studies have shown no relationship between diet and migraine headaches.

Such statements help us to understand one of the rules of orthodox medicine. Before you receive a treatment, it must generally speaking have been 'proven' effective against a particular disease, by means of clinical trials. If no trials have been carried out, or if the trial methodology was not considered 'rigorous' enough, or if the study wasn't carried out at a recognized institution, or if the results didn't get into one of the major medical journals, or if some of the trials that have been carried out showed that it worked, and others showed that it didn't, the treatment is considered 'unproven' and your doctor is unlikely to prescribe it. So although he or she might have read somewhere about a physiological connection between chocolate and migraine headaches, your doctor is more likely to give you painkillers than to suggest that you try avoiding chocolate and other foods linked with the same problem. Most doctors do not even bother to inform their patients of the known connection between chocolate and migraine.

On the surface this sounds reasonable enough. After all, if a new drug was being developed and a clinical trial showed that it didn't work, it would not be allowed on the market. All drugs are toxic, and some are highly dangerous. The approval of every drug is dependent on its proven risk:benefit ratio. That is to say the answer to the question: 'Do the benefits of this drug outweigh its toxicity and side effects?'

But when we come to nutritional treatments it is not a reasonable approach at all. In nutritional treatments we are taking away substances which are hindering the efficiency of an individual's biological function, and repleting the individual with substances which that individual is lacking.

It would be about as logical to expect every group of migraine patients to react badly to chocolate, as it would be to expect every group of PMS sufferers to respond favourably to vitamin B_6 or evening primrose oil supplements. Yet this is

PRINCIPLES OF NUTRITIONAL THERAPY

what the orthodox world expects from a nutritional treatment, and it is the reason why you will not get nutritional therapy (as defined in this book) from a conventional doctor or dietitian, despite the fact that so much of this therapy has firm scientific foundations based on knowledge of physiology, biochemistry and function.

Even a television set has the right to an investigation into the cause of faulty function. Repair engineers do not give all broken-down TV sets (with the same problem) the same new spare part. Yet, broadly speaking, this is the basis of modern medicine. It may seem incredible, but it is perfectly true.

Most people don't know this, and assume that if they had a biological abnormality then their doctor would pick up on it. But doctors are not picking up on the abnormalities that I describe in this book. Doctors do not carry out routine tests for nutritional deficiency on PMS sufferers or eczema sufferers. They do not test for hypochlorhydria in people with bloating and indigestion, or leaky gut in people with multiple food sensitivities. They do not test for pesticides or carry out liver function tests on patients with chronic fatigue or asthma, or test a migraine sufferer's ability to process tyramine and phenylethylamine, or carry out glucose tolerance tests on people with depression and mood swings. For these people, who in many cases are already eating a healthy diet, conventional nutritional advice does not help. And the drug treatments which are administered at enormous expense will never get to the root of the problem and will probably cause metabolic abnormalities of their own. Worst of all, many patients who have protested that drug treatments are ineffective or cause unacceptable side effects, know only too well that they may receive very unsympathetic treatment, or even a psychiatric referral, from their doctor.

WHAT HAPPENS WHEN YOU CONSULT A NUTRITIONAL THERAPIST?

Treating a person (as opposed to a disease) means finding out what their individual needs are and how to fulfil them.

Determining someone's needs involves carrying out a diagnostic procedure. Our patient may tell us that he/she has already been given a diagnosis: for instance 'asthma' or 'psoriasis'. But in complementary medicine, diagnosis means identifying needs, not diseases.

The nutritional therapist would ideally like to send each patient for a battery of tests to assess the status of 30 different nutrients, to test for food allergies, heavy metal toxicity, chemical sensitivities, gut permeability, gut parasitology, nutrient malabsorption, glucose tolerance, liver function, hypochlorhydria, pancreatic function, and so on. Unfortunately the cost for most people would be prohibitive since it may not be reimbursable under insurance schemes or national health schemes, especially if the practitioner is not a qualified doctor.

The nutritional therapist can, however, often make a working diagnosis on the basis of symptom analysis. In fact this can sometimes be a more sensitive method of diagnosis. I once had a patient who had been seriously ill with multiple allergies for many years. She was so chemically sensitive that she almost lost consciousness in the presence of tobacco smoke. This in itself told me that her body was not detoxifying properly and was overloaded with toxins. Her history of many courses of antibiotics and very resistant vaginal thrush strongly suggested the presence of intestinal or even systemic candidiasis, which could be a significant contributor to her toxic overload, so I initiated treatment for this immediately. Her symptoms also suggested a number of nutritional deficiencies, particularly B vitamins, zinc and magnesium, and I gave her supplements of these. With this regime and a hypoallergenic diet, she began to make progress for the first time.

It turned out that this lady (who was a psychologist) had earlier consulted a well-known doctor in the nutritional therapy movement who proceeded to have a number of tests carried out for her. On the basis of the results of these tests, he sent her away as 'completely healthy and as strong as a horse'. Needless to say, she was extremely angry at yet another doctor refusing to listen to her, and the waste of her money.

METHODS

The nutritional therapist almost always begins with a detailed questionnaire which the patient fills in before the first appointment. This saves a great deal of time, since the therapist can skim quickly through it and pick out those areas which require further questioning. Sometimes the patient simply puts his or her medical diagnosis down on the questionnaire and then the therapist must ask exactly what symptoms are experienced. This is because diagnoses like 'irritable bowel syndrome' may cover a great many combinations of symptoms, such as bloating, diarrhoea, constipation, pain, flatulence, discomfort, each of which varies from one patient to the next and suggests different factors involved in the causation of the bowel problem.

Questions include those on condition of skin, eyes and fingernails, energy levels, mood, nerves, pain, menstrual and premenstrual symptoms (for women), sleep, digestion, frequency of bowel movements, presence of mucus, health history, current medications, diet, stress, exercise and exposure to pollution. Knowledge of the patient's full spectrum of symptoms, from split fingernails to constipation is essential for the nutritional therapist, no matter how irrelevant these symptoms may appear to be. The body has a reason for each one, and the therapist is trying to build up a picture of what is going wrong

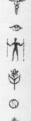

PRINCIPLES OF NUTRITIONAL THERAPY

internally. Details of the patient's lifestyle can also help to explain their current condition.

EXAMPLES OF DIAGNOSES

VERONICA

Veronica, aged 19, came to me because she wanted to lose weight. After completing her questionnaire, it was revealed that she suffered from extreme fatigue, finding it an effort to walk 200 yards to her nearest bus-stop. She ate only hamburgers and chips (which she craved) and breakfast cereal. My diagnosis: nutritional deficiencies. I gave her multivitamins/minerals and some simple advice on how to cook nutritious vegetable soups, which she was to eat in large quantities. (She had never cooked before, and didn't know how to.) Veronica lost 7 lb without difficulty, regained her energy and also lost her craving for hamburger and chips.

JANE

Jane, aged 28 and with one small daughter, came to me with a doctor's diagnosis of rheumatoid arthritis. Her questionnaire revealed a multitude of symptoms: joint pains, headaches, diarrhoea alternating with constipation, fatigue, sinusitis and skin rashes. My diagnosis: food allergy. A hypoallergenic diet was prescribed (with multivitamins and digestive enzymes), which cleared up her symptoms. After a period of challenge testing we identified milk and dairy produce as the offending foods.

MICHAEL

Michael had suffered from digestive difficulties for some months and a pain in his liver, made a great deal worse by eating fatty food. The doctor offered to remove his gall bladder. Michael refused. My diagnosis: liver or gall-bladder congestion

causing food sensitivity. I gave Michael digestive enzymes,
liver decongestant herbs and a diet cutting out all meat, dairy
produce and saturated fat, to lighten the load on his digestion.
But he was allowed nuts (which contain a lot of oil) and extra
virgin olive oil. He tolerated the diet very well and the tender-
ness around his liver gradually disappeared.

JOAN

Joan, aged 62, had been given very strong antidepressant drugs
for what had been diagnosed as clinical depression. She particularly wanted help with an unusual symptom: she would fall
asleep as soon as she was sitting in a relaxed position, in a the-
atre, cinema or at home reading the newspaper. These naps felt
to her like a 'coma' and after waking she felt extremely ill. My
diagnosis: possibly a reaction to the drugs. A basic diagnostic
diet was administered, which helped a great deal. After further
work it was discovered that sugar consumption considerably
aggravated the problem.

AGNES

Agnes, aged 60, came to me because her doctor had told her to
lose weight. However, she was already on a very low-calorie
diet. My diagnosis: fluid retention due to an adverse reaction to
beta blocker drugs prescribed for her blood pressure, causing
excess weight. I suggested that Agnes return to her doctor to
explain that she had only gained weight after starting the
drugs, to show him her puffy ankles and to force him to believe
that she was already on a low-calorie diet.

Building up a picture of how a person's health has become
undermined requires finding out as much about them as
possible.

EXAMPLE:

AUDREY

For five years Audrey, aged 29, had suffered from icy cold extremities even in the warmest weather, facial hot flushes, muscular tension and extreme insomnia, none of which symptoms in themselves suggested any particular nutritional diagnosis. She was very health conscious, and her diet consisted of fish, vegetables, fruit, salads, brown rice and beans, carefully cooked. She took multivitamins and minerals daily, and I could not identify any particular indicators of nutritional deficiency, except perhaps magnesium. Magnesium is needed for good circulation, muscle relaxation and sleep. Audrey herself had already identified intolerances to wheat and dairy produce, which gave her assorted symptoms like headaches and bowel upsets. She did not seem to have any further allergies.

An experienced nutritional therapist knows at this point that the clue to the problem very possibly lies in the answer to the question: 'What happened five years ago when the problems started?'

Audrey had been working on her family's farm, in the large greenhouses. Her job was to spray the plants with pesticide. Due to the very hot weather, her face and arms were bare as she did this work, and no one suggested that she might need a protective mask.

Audrey sprayed and sprayed all summer. But it was not until some months after the work stopped that her symptoms began to develop. She had never associated them with the spraying. Her doctor administered various drugs, but there was no real relief from the problems.

Pesticides are neurotoxins, designed to damage the nervous system of any living creature that comes into contact with them. Once we had pieced together this history, Audrey's symptoms were really not all that surprising.

Work began on Audrey, using increased amounts of nutrients that are normally used as raw materials to help eliminate toxic substances from the body. Audrey also needed to take as many saunas as possible, to help sweat the poisons out through her skin. Finally she began to make progress and her insomnia started to ease. What also helped greatly was the reduction in the (perfectly natural) anxiety which she had experienced for so long because she didn't know what was wrong with her. Many sick people experience this alleviation of anxiety after consulting a complementary medicine practitioner, from a sense of relief that someone is finally in charge again and has a plan of action. The therapeutic effect of this cannot be doubted, but it is a contribution to the healing process, not the sole factor responsible.

The nutritional therapist takes many factors into account when forming a diagnosis. Even events in babyhood such as rashes or diarrhoea which later cleared up can be significant, indicating a possible history of food allergy, for instance. The present diet can give clues to the cause of symptoms, but so can the past diet, which was being followed when the symptoms first began and may have led to the development of nutritional deficiencies, the effects of which have not yet been overcome.

Stress is assessed, so that those patients whose symptoms are most likely to be primarily stress-related can be identified and referred for help elsewhere. Exercise habits are examined, and also exposure to toxic substances in the home or at work.

MOSTAPHA: A CASE OF CHRONIC FATIGUE

Mostapha, a fast food restaurant chef, was referred to me by a doctor for chronic fatigue. Mostapha was very distressed about the problem, since he needed to support his young family, but could barely struggle through a day's work.

After asking some routine questions, I discovered that

Mostapha did have some periods of relief from his fatigue, particularly on his days off and on holiday. It quickly became clear that Mostapha's symptoms were connected with his place of work. I asked if any chemicals were in use, and he recalled sometimes feeling particularly ill when the toilets had just been cleaned and the smell of the cleaning fluid wafted into the kitchen.

It seemed very likely that Mostapha was suffering from some form of chemical sensitivity. The cleaning fluid was changed and Mostapha's symptoms cleared up.

Each of the cases mentioned in this chapter were successfully treated. But the success was due to identifying each individual person's needs. We cannot cure all cases of rheumatoid arthritis by removing milk from the diet. We cannot cure all insomnia by supporting liver function, or all cases of tiredness by changing the patient's toilet cleaner and we shall probably never cure anyone else's 'coma' again by removing sugar!

Trends in medicine come and go, and the present preoccupation with nutritional research that gives a single treatment formula to all patients with a particular Western diagnosis for a finite and defined time will eventually be seen as inappropriate and obstructive to progress.

AFTER DIAGNOSIS

Diagnosis in nutritional therapy is always tentative at first, and the initial diagnosis is a so-called 'working' diagnosis, for the purpose of designing a therapeutic trial. A therapeutic trial is an experimental regime which is calculated to be likely to result in therapeutic benefit.

So a patient diagnosed as being a likely candidate for food allergy or intolerance will be given a hypoallergenic diagnostic diet to test out this theory. This is a diet excluding all the foods which most often cause reactions in allergic or sensitive people, as well as ingredients which contain these foods in hidden form. It is administered for two weeks to see whether symptoms are relieved. If so, the symptoms were probably allergic in origin.

But nutritional therapy is a holistic treatment, and not just concerned with identifying problem foods and sending someone away again with instructions to avoid them. Allergy is a sign of malfunction in the body, and the nutritional therapist would feel that he or she is not doing their job properly if they did not take measures to improve function and prevent a further deterioration in health, which might perhaps lead to further allergies.

So the initial diagnostic diet will usually also exclude foods which in some way stress the body or force it to work harder. These include tea, coffee and chocolate because of their content of caffeine and other methylxanthines (natural chemicals linked with fibrocystic breast disease, for example), alcohol, salt and salted foods, sugar, red meat and saturated fat. The patient is encouraged to use only fresh, whole foods.

For suspected allergy sufferers the nutritional therapist will usually also prescribe digestive enzyme supplements and supplements or herbs which promote intestinal health, since the development of an allergy is thought to be linked with the leakage of partially digested food particles through an over-permeable gut wall.

The effect of this type of diagnostic diet is often remarkably positive. Some seriously ill people will have to remain on it on a long-term basis, but others can soon be put through a challenge testing procedure to determine which foods are symptom-inducing, and may then graduate to a less stringent 'maintenance' diet (see page 128).

Challenge testing must be carried out very carefully under expert guidance. There are a number of different types of

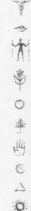

allergic reaction: immediate, delayed, intermittent, and those requiring multiple exposure. There are also life-threatening allergic reactions, and individuals who already know that they have dangerous responses to peanuts, for example, must never try to undertake challenge testing on such foods.

Allergic reactions can be deceptive, and can change. For instance certain food supplements can result in the disappearance of headaches as an allergic symptom, and a food challenge will no longer cause headaches. But the pain of the headaches may have previously masked a simultaneous feeling of 'brain fag', which still remains. If this occurs after food challenge, the sufferer may not realize that it is an allergic reaction, especially if it is delayed.

The nutritional therapist's programme of food challenge testing will normally last for about six weeks and a maintenance diet will then be prescribed, the aim of which is to keep the individual feeling as healthy as possible while fitting as well as possible into their lifestyle. During this six-week period the therapist will work much teaching about health and nutrition into the therapy sessions, for instance explaining the detailed workings of the digestive system and intestines, some of the causes of their dysfunction, and how the treatment programme is designed to address these factors. Since the patient's co-operation is essential, it is more likely to be obtained if the patient fully understands the reasons for everything that he or she is asked to do, and can visualize the effects of the treatment on the internal organs. Some patients come away having learned much simple physiology and biochemistry, which they find fascinating and, together with the improvement in their symptoms, makes them determined never to maltreat their body again.

Simple allergies and nutritional deficiencies are easy to treat in this way. Once symptoms improve they generally continue to do so. Once the point can be reached where a simple maintenance programme is adequate for the patient's needs, the patient can be sent off to continue improving without further regular supervision.

Some severe chronic illnesses such as myalgic encephalomyelitis (ME) are much more difficult to deal with. The most common problem which nutritional therapists face from such patients is impatience. After the initial improvement in symptoms (which usually occurs after the removal of allergenic problem foods) the ME sufferer despairs when the inevitable plateau is reached: the point at which progress is no longer rapid and improvements are more readily seen by outsiders who don't have regular contact with the patient, than the patients themselves. It is very difficult to explain to a bedbound, semi-paralysed ME sufferer that without nutritional therapy it may often take as long as eight years to get better, but that even with nutritional therapy it may take two years. Most of my ME patients have given up after four to six months because the improvements in weakness and fatigue were not rapid enough for them. If they decide to continue taking dietary supplements, they may just buy one or two products that they have read about (like vitamin C and evening primrose oil), or else buy whatever is the latest fad in the ME community.

ME and other degenerative diseases like arthritis, cancers and Alzheimer's disease, ideally require both vigorous detoxification work on the body and raw materials for the rebuilding and repair of damaged functions. Individual diet programmes usually have to be formulated, and many dietary supplements and herbal products will usually be needed. These will not remain the same throughout the treatment programme, as is sometimes assumed, but will change as the therapist addresses different priorities in a structured programme.

Rose, aged 82, had had osteoarthritis since her late 30s and had recently been diagnosed with osteoporosis, for which her doctor had prescribed two pints of milk a day and calcium tablets. A diagnostic diet revealed that much of Rose's joint pain was allergy-related, and the spinal pain, which was not, could be mostly relieved by a back support device called a Back Friend (see Appendix II for where to obtain these). This is a wonderful device which consists of a rigid seat and rigid shaped back support, hinged together, which can be carried around and placed on soft seats such as car seats. The support which it gives to both the upper and lower back affords much relief to those with spinal problems.

Rose's allergies were in fact milk and yeast (the doctor's prescribed milk had made her much worse) and these had also caused her 40 years of severe bloating and intestinal malabsorption. So our first task was to give her digestive soothing agents like the herb slippery elm, as well as comfrey, liquorice, fennel, peppermint, chamomile and marshmallow herbal teas. Vitamin U (a substance extracted from cabbage with proven gut healing properties) was administered as a supplement, as well as vitamins and minerals to help make good the deficiencies from which she was likely to be suffering.

Next we moved the emphasis to work on Rose's liver function, and gave her a programme of herbs and dietary supplements to help her eliminate toxic substances which had probably been readily absorbed through her dysfunctional intestinal walls for too long. These were thought to be the cause of her residual aches and pains, although the osteoporosis might also be responsible.

Finally we worked to give priority support to nourishing Rose's bones, using ground up comfrey leaves (an excellent tissue strengthener), boron, magnesium (which is often more important than calcium), mineral supplements, vitamin D and a herbal formula to support the parathyroid glands, which are involved in the absorption and excretion of calcium.

Despite her age, Rose became virtually pain-free within about six months, unless she over-exerted herself, and our task was next to build up her muscles, atrophied because of so many years' reduced mobility due to arthritic pain. Exercise is one of the most important factors for the prevention of osteoporosis, and we hoped that, even if our treatment might not result in improving Rose's bone density, we could at least prevent the osteoporosis from getting worse.

It was a great disappointment that Rose would not tell her doctor about her nutritional treatment and its great success. She was afraid he would be angry that she had consulted an alternative practitioner. This is sadly only too true for most patients. No doubt he believes to this day that her improvement was due to his prescription of milk and calcium.

Nutritional therapy is a dynamic treatment – it establishes an order of priority and then tackles each of these priorities in turn, seeking to enhance different aspects of health during the process. As one function begins to improve, this in turn affects other functions, and, just as the spiral of downward health has a downward 'domino' effect on biological functions, the reverse happens as these functions recover.

There are, of course, many tragic cases where nutritional therapy, even when used as part of a holistic programme, does not result in recovery from a serious chronic illness. No reputable practitioner would ever claim to guarantee a cure. Seriously ill patients should approach this therapy as they would approach the subject of car maintenance. A car cannot run at full efficiency if it is given poor quality fuel, or if the fuel cannot get to where it is needed, or the mechanisms are clogged up with waste matter. In this respect, the body's disease-fighting functions are very similar.

STRESS

A good nutritional therapist will not just consider nutritional factors. An equally important contributor to illness is stress. When I work with patients my alarm bells start sounding very loudly when someone comes into my consulting room in a state of anxiety.

One case in particular comes to mind. A housewife (let's call her Angela) consulted me for what she had self-diagnosed as candidiasis. Her main symptom was fatigue. She was also generally unwell and depressed.

Although Angela had consulted me for a nutritional programme, I felt that this was the last thing she needed just at present. It is particularly important to remember that a difficult nutritional programme can greatly add to stress, and the therapist should be conscious of this at all times. Angela's diet was reasonably good, and she was already taking a multivitamin, so her most basic nutritional needs were taken care of.

One of the most important rules in any form of medicine is 'prioritization': dealing first of all with what is the most obvious. There was an air of hysteria around Angela when she walked into my consulting room. Her inner tension was so great that her speech was speeded up and high-pitched, she could not focus or concentrate on anything except her anxiety about her symptoms, and it was clear that if she went on this way something would snap. Clearly what she expected from me was that, after writing down all her symptoms, I would come up with a diet which would finally destroy this yeast on which she blamed her lack of energy to cope with the stresses in her life.

But I could see that if Angela was tired it was more than likely that it was not the fatigue which was causing her stress, but vice versa. I stopped her in mid-flow and explained that before I could give her any nutritional advice I needed her to be in a calmer state of mind. She hardly heard me, and it was clear that she was in no state to take in anything very much. I repeated that I could not help her while she was so fraught. Finally she allowed me to carry out a short relaxation exercise with her, using a little guided imagery to slow down her heart rate and breathing, stop her flood of anxious thoughts and give her a chance to connect with me on a different level, putting herself in my hands rather than taking control of the therapy session herself. I often do a little hands-on healing with people like this. I just rest my hands on their shoulders from behind, and this aids a sense of calmness and peace. Many people can do this if they have inner peace themselves, and you too may wish to try it on friends, loved ones or patients in times of distress.

There was a remarkable change in Angela once she had relinquished control to me. She was now able to listen and absorb information, the tension, now gone, had obviously been holding in her despair. I asked Angela about the stresses in her life and without hesitation she began to describe the horror story of her marriage. In a nutshell, Angela was being subjected to emotional torture from her husband, who would not stop his violent verbal attacks on almost everything she did, in which he was supported by his mother, who lived with them. Angela's confidence in herself was non-existent, and she had no one to give her moral and emotional support. She wanted very much to leave her husband, but had nowhere else to go for herself and her son. She wept as she described how she felt completely trapped.

This was a difficult problem indeed, and I knew that Angela would not survive for very long unless she sought help from a counsellor. She needed to have someone on her side who could help her truly understand that her husband's verbal attacks were the product of a disturbed mind and were not an accurate reflection of how she really was. I explained that counselling might not change her situation, but that it could change her reaction to it. It was this reaction which was causing her so much pain.

Angela saw the sense of this and her spirits were visibly lifted and strengthened, which happens with everyone who feels helpless and then finds a way to take action. In itself it is very therapeutic. I told Angela to come back and see me if she felt she still needed a nutritional programme after consulting a counsellor. She never did, and I hope that she is making progress.

Complementary medicine is often accused of only producing results because its practitioners spend more time with patients, helping them to feel better by listening to their worries and anxieties. Oddly enough our critics say this as if they think we don't realize the therapeutic effect of listening. It is only too unfortunate that so many of them don't follow our example. They might learn a great deal.

ANOTHER KIND OF STRESS

Every nutritional therapist has experienced the kind of patient who makes an appointment on the understanding that nutritional therapy isn't going to take up much of their time with cooking, because they are too busy to spend time in the kitchen!

We all know the type. They are often executives, work hard and play hard, have a hectic social life and lots of commitments which frequently involve ingesting copious amounts of alcohol. A lack of time for mundane matters is held as a status symbol. A typical case might feel under par for some time, block it out because that's their usual way of coping with everything, keep up the same lifestyle, and then come down with a more serious health problem which makes them realize something must be done. This type (which I normally refer to as 'physically stressed') usually believes that something quite simple and minimally inconvenient can sort them out, like eating more carrots or taking a vitamin that they haven't discovered yet. They are products of the 'instant' era. Instant coffee, instant food, instant entertainment, instant medicines, instant service, computers that perform tasks instantly. There must be a way to cheat nature and obtain instant health.

Unfortunately there isn't. As the ancient Spanish proverb says, 'Take what you want, and pay for it.' The root cause of any health problems suffered by the physically stressed type is not so much diet but attitude, a lack of concern for their body. Coffee, cigarettes and booze, late nights, driving their body constantly to the point of exhaustion, rushing to meet deadlines, to beat the traffic, to beat the competition, to take on other people's problems, all this takes its toll and wear and tear is the result. For some it comes sooner than for others.

The difficulty in treatment comes when you ask someone like this to change the amount of physical stress to which they subject themselves. I often get a look which says: 'stick to diet please, that's what I'm paying you for.' It is very difficult to explain to someone who doesn't know how to unwind completely, who is so out of tune with their body that they don't notice its warning signals, that natural medicine isn't about a 'quick fix' to get you back on the road with the minimum disruption to your timetable. It is about understanding that the body is a separate entity from the will or mind, that it has needs of its own, and that it must be treated with the same consideration that you would treat a friend whom you love.

So when Jenny, a physically stressed type, returned for her two-week follow-up after starting the health programme I set her, I wasn't surprised when she said that she hadn't actually started the diet yet because she didn't have time to go shopping. She had, however, cut down on coffee and wine. I met with a blank stare when I enquired how she had got on with my instructions for rest and relaxation, as if to say 'with a busy schedule like mine how can I possibly have time for that!'

However, all is not lost, even with a client like Jenny. It is part of the nutritional therapist's job to cope with clients who need extra motivation. So when I receive a response like this, I usually reply, 'How can you expect your body to keep performing for you when you keep taking from it all the time and never give anything back?'

Jenny thought profoundly about what I had said, and from then on began to work towards listening to her body. Resting when she was tired, learning that it was OK not to be hectic all the time, and beginning to revolve her life around her body's needs rather than the other way round.

Of course her new attitude calmed her down a lot, which was therapeutic in itself, and we were soon able to work on her diet, which sorted out the headaches from which she had regularly suffered. It was in fact the large amounts of coffee she had been drinking (in order to keep up with her frantic lifestyle) which had been responsible for her headaches.

Not every case is so successful. In some individuals physical stress is so much part of their lives that they simply cannot get out of its treadmill. I refer such cases for autogenic training (see Appendix II), a type of therapy which teaches a meditative state of mind in order to get back in tune with the body.

SOME COMMON ILLNESSES FROM THE NUTRITIONAL THERAPIST'S VIEW

Because they are not usually trained in orthodox medical diagnosis, all reputable nutritional therapists prefer their patients to consult a doctor first, and also to maintain contact with their doctor in case orthodox treatment becomes advisable or necessary (such as in cases of diabetes, bowel obstruction, or a need for tumour excision, for example). It is the complementary medicine practitioner's aim that the patient should have the best of both worlds, not to take the place of necessary orthodox medical care.

A doctor's medical diagnosis can also contribute to the nutritional therapist's understanding of how to approach an individual patient. Much nutritional research has been carried out into specific illnesses, and the known physiology and biochemistry of these illnesses can help to suggest useful avenues to pursue.

AIDS

This disease results in a severely compromised digestive system, and multiple nutritional problems are acknowledged to be common, as well as candidiasis, which is due to the malfunction of the immune system. One nutritional deficiency that receives scant attention is selenium, now thought to be specifically depleted by HIV.

There is increasing evidence that Aids is really an auto-immune disease, in which the immune system attacks its own cells which, due to HIV, are no longer recognizable as 'self'. As with other similarly serious diseases, all that the nutritional therapist can do for the sufferer is to seek ways to encourage good function, using the basic principles of nutritional therapy. The earlier the HIV+ individual consults the nutritional therapist, the better, in the hope of halting or at worst slowing down, any progression to full-blown Aids.

ALZHEIMER'S DISEASE
AND SENILE DEMENTIA

A number of different nutritional deficiencies are thought to be common in dementia sufferers, including B vitamins, zinc and magnesium. Severe deficiencies of folic acid or vitamin B_3, for example, are known causes of dementia, and the elderly are a recognized risk group for malnourishment due to apathy from living alone, worsening digestion and absorption as age progresses, and sometimes poorly-fitting dentures.

There also seems to be a link between aluminium in drinking water and the incidence of Alzheimer's disease, and aluminium has been found in the brains of Alzheimer's patients. A deficiency of zinc or magnesium can encourage the assimilation of aluminium.

One cause of Alzheimer's disease is thought to be large numbers of tiny clots in the blood supply to the brain, causing many 'mini-strokes'.

The nutritional therapist will consider these factors and also work towards enhancing liver function to aid the elimination of toxic substances that may be damaging brain function.

Nutritional therapy is ideally suited to help improve the blood circulation to the brain and to prevent clot formation.

ARTHRITIS

Arthritis simply means 'joint pain'. Food intolerances, certain types of nutritional deficiency, and a toxic overload can result in joint pain, among other symptoms. Some of the causes of osteoarthritis which have been identified in different sufferers are:

- Intolerance to red meat and saturated fat.

- Intolerance to common food allergens (eg wheat, yeast, dairy produce, food additives).

- Deficiencies of EPA or GLA, which are produced within the body from oils in the diet (EPA is also found in oily fish like sardines). Production can be inhibited by alcohol consumption and by deficiencies of zinc, vitamin B_6 and magnesium.

- Excess tissue acidity.

- Constipation.

Rheumatoid arthritis is an auto-immune disease. It is often linked with food allergies, but there are usually other components and it can be much more difficult to improve than osteoarthritis.

ASTHMA

Doctors acknowledge that asthma is often linked with inhalant allergies such as to house dust mite and animals, but they rarely accept food allergy as a cause of symptoms. In the experience of nutritional therapists this chronic condition is the result of a complex breakdown of health which frequently involves nutritional deficiencies, food allergies and a toxic overload and can in many cases be improved by addressing these factors.

BIRTH DEFECTS

Mainstream medicine now sees gene therapy as the future solution to birth defects, and there is plenty of funding to research this technologically satisfying avenue of experimentation. Medicine is hardly even noticing the researchers who have linked birth defects with nutritional deficiencies and excesses of toxic heavy metals like cadmium and lead. Dr Neil Ward at Surrey University in England is a leading researcher in this field, working with extraordinarily little funding with the organization Foresight, a charity for preconceptional care. Researchers Margaret and Arthur Wynn, also lone voices in their field, believe that if everybody had a proper intake of fresh vegetables, fruit, nuts and seeds, mutations leading to problems like Downs syndrome could in time be eradicated.

Deficiencies of folic acid and zinc have been most strongly linked with abnormal foetal development. It is extraordinary that the acceptance of folic acid supplementation as a preventive treatment for spina bifida, has not led to concern about nutritional deficiency as a potential cause of birth defects. Instead folic acid is seen as an 'anti spina bifida drug' and is given in massive doses to many pregnant women instead of simply ensuring that their diet is adequate.

Pesticides and other toxic chemicals may also be involved in birth defects. For instance there have been outbreaks of babies born without eyes in some areas where there is more intensive

CANCERS

In *A Cancer Therapy: Results of Fifty Cases*, nutritional therapy pioneer Dr Max Gerson writes:

> In my opinion cancer is not a problem of deficiencies in hormones, vitamins and enzymes. It is not a problem of allergies or infections with a virus or any other known or unknown microorganism. It is not a poisoning through some special intermediary metabolic substance or any other substance coming from the outside – so-called carcinogenic substances. All these can be partial causative agents in man ... Cancer is ... an accumulation of numerous damaging factors combined in deteriorating the whole metabolism, after the liver has been progressively impaired in its functions.

Science has consistently rejected Max Gerson's therapy, while in fact gradually coming into line with his thinking. The Gerson diet, with its emphasis on juices made from leafy green vegetables, is a rich source of antioxidants and indoles which assist cytochrome P450 oxidase enzymes in the liver, now known to be important in neutralizing both carcinogens and excess hormones.

Cancer is thought to occur when carcinogenic substances damage the nucleus of a cell. They do this by producing free oxidizing radicals, rogue oxygen molecules which seek to combine with molecules within living tissues, causing much damage in the process.

The cell nucleus contains the genetic or 'blueprint' material for a cell, the instructions which ensure that when it reproduces, the new cells will be 'differentiated', that is to say that

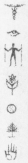

they will function as they should. But as Dr Nadya Coates explains in *A Matter of Life*:

> If the cell nucleus is damaged, bits of genetic material can ooze out ... It is a law of life that as soon as there is even a bit of a gene, every piece 'wants' to become a cell and to become a nucleus, but it would do so without the full genetic information required for a cell to reach differentiation and maturity.

Such cells instead form 'tumours', tissues which proliferate abnormally, do not behave as normal body tissue, and, if malignant, can interfere with normal body function and spread to other parts of the body.

The immune system of a healthy body detects and destroys such aberrant cells before they can form tumours. So for cancers to form, the body must already be to some extent unhealthy. Nutritional therapy seeks to encourage healthy function and, although it is much more difficult for the immune system to destroy a full-blown tumour rather than just a few aberrant cells, it has happened many times, and some very advanced cases of cancer have returned to complete health. Such cases are referred to as 'natural remissions', and patients who have experienced them have attributed them to a variety of different causes, including change in diet and use of dietary supplements (particularly vitamin C megadoses); reduction of stress; finding new enjoyment and meaning in life, perhaps through psychotherapy or religion; 'deciding' to or willing oneself to get well; visualizing the immune system winning over the cancer cells; and the use of a spiritual healer.

Cancer is a disease in which emotional and psychological stress, and the sense of a lack of fulfilment in life can play an enormously important part in depressing the immune system. In these cases a good nutritional therapist will not add to the stress by imposing a difficult dietary regime immediately, but will work gently towards promoting good health, while encouraging the individual to seek counselling or psychotherapy.

Vitamin C therapy is a particularly important part of nutritional therapy for cancer. It is surprising that orthodox doctors rarely suggest that their patients take vitamin C supplements since there is much research to show that it is non-toxic even in extremely high doses, and increases the number, size and motility of the white blood cells which fight cancer. Both human and animal studies have demonstrated that with long-term use it can also increase survival time. In my opinion it is very wrong to withhold such information from cancer patients. If they have to find it out for themselves, they can only lose faith in their doctor.

CHRONIC FATIGUE AND MYALGIC ENCEPHALOMYELITIS (ME)

This is not one disease but is the end result of severe damage to the body's energy-production mechanisms, by whatever means this may be. Research shows that factors such as a history of vaccination and much antibiotic use often seem to be involved in the development of ME. Some severe cases have been described as 'atypical polio'. Vaccination introduces micro-organisms such as the polio virus into the body which might not otherwise be there, and it is thought that these may in later life, if the individual becomes particularly run down, proliferate and cause damage to the body.

Liver detoxification pathways are commonly severely impaired in ME sufferers, who are intolerant of alcohol and medications, both of which must be detoxified by the liver. Many so-called 'ME' patients admitted to environmental

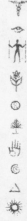

medicine units have been found to be really victims of environmental and occupational poisoning, such as from sheep dip, other types of pesticide exposure and industrial chemicals and pollutants.

Nutritional deficiencies, allergies and a toxic overload are all common in ME sufferers, who, according to a study carried out by the British charity Action for ME, report that 'diet and supplements' is the most effective treatment. Some cases respond to nutritional therapy within a few weeks; others take a year or more.

EATING DISORDERS

Although nutritional deficiencies such as zinc have been implicated in some cases of anorexia nervosa, both this and bulimia nervosa are primarily psychological disorders centring around issues of 'control'. Anorexics and bulimics may consult alternative nutritional therapists, but unless they have had successful psychotherapy, this is really only because they do not want to put on weight and are hoping that the nutritional therapist will tell them that the sugar and fatty foods which their dietitian has prescribed are unhealthy and should not be eaten. Naturally for anorexia nervosa this is not true and such foods should be eaten in large amounts until the patient's body weight normalizes. The nutritional therapist should refer such cases to specialist centres or organizations dealing with eating disorders and perhaps also suggest a useful psychological therapy such as Eriksonian hypnotherapy (See Appendix II).

EPILEPSY

Epilepsy is a serious disease which is generally of unknown cause, but its onset is becoming increasingly linked with exposure to pesticides. However, proper research is yet to be done because victims are hesitant to come forward. A diagnosis of epilepsy means the withdrawal of a driving licence and possibly a loss of livelihood since farm tenancies may be conditional upon good health.

Allergic people may suffer epileptic seizures as an allergic symptom. They may not be aware of the role of allergy in their illness, or that they can prevent seizures by identifying and avoiding allergens.

Seizures can also occur in the presence of a severe vitamin B_6, zinc or magnesium deficiency, or a vitamin B_6 dependency (see page 29 for an explanation of vitamin dependency).

GALL BLADDER DISEASE

Gallstones are linked with a poor diet, in particular an excess of saturated fat and sugar and a lack of dietary fibre. A number of foods and dietary supplements can help to increase the solubility of bile, which is the liquid found in the gall bladder, in time helping to dissolve gall stones. Meanwhile the nutritional therapist can usually work with the patient to find a diet which keeps him/her reasonably pain-free. (A fat-free diet, sometimes prescribed by dietitians, is not the answer since this encourages gall bladder stagnation.) If the stones are small enough, the nutritional therapist may be able to prescribe a gall bladder 'flush' treatment which ejects them and enables them to be eliminated via the stools.

HEART DISEASE

Heart disease was rare until relatively recently. Medical historians pass off our present epidemic as a natural consequence of living longer, but the great increase in our average life

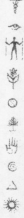

expectancy is due mainly to a reduction in infant deaths. Even in the early twentieth century if you made it past infancy you had quite a good chance of living out your 'three score years and ten'.

Heart disease occurs when the coronary artery becomes narrowed with cholesterol deposits and can no longer carry an adequate blood supply to the heart. The deposition of cholesterol on the artery walls is encouraged by dietary factors, particularly a diet high in saturated fat and low in fibre. Magnesium deficiency can cause artery spasms leading to a dangerous temporary narrowing of the artery. An EPA deficiency can lead to excessive 'stickiness' of the blood, which promotes the formation of clots which can block the arteries. Food allergies can cause severe fluid retention which increases the volume of blood and therefore encourages high blood pressure, dangerous for those with heart disease.

Nutritional therapy is ideally suited to addressing these risk factors, and in time can even gradually reduce blood cholesterol levels and strip cholesterol deposits from the walls of the coronary artery, thus reducing the narrowing of the artery and the attendant angina pain which occurs on exertion.

In 1994 *Nutritional Therapy Today*, the journal of the Society for the Promotion of Nutritional Therapy in the UK (see Appendix II), reported the case of David Holmes, a former severe angina sufferer who had been able to come off all angina and heart medication after following a nutritional therapy regime for only ten months. From being able to walk only a few yards, he progressed to climbing mountains in his spare time.

INFERTILITY

The UK organization Foresight (see Appendix II) specializes in the natural treatment of infertility, and has identified poor diet,

JOHN SMITH
& SON

YOU'LL
DISCOVER
IT ALL

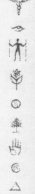

nutritional deficiencies, a toxic overload, hidden infections and
many other factors as potential causes of infertility. In particular vitamin C or zinc deficiency can reduce the quantity and/or motility of sperm in the male partner. Researchers Margaret and Arthur Wynn have identified numerous common foods, medicines and other factors which cause mutations in both eggs and sperm. Up to 50 per cent of miscarriages are in fact due to poor quality sperm in the male partner according to Swedish research.

IRRITABLE BOWEL SYNDROME

This is a condition involving discomfort and dysfunction in the lower intestinal tract, and nutritional therapists will look at each symptom reported by the individual sufferer and try to determine the cause. The most common causes are stress, food intolerance and poor digestion. Some practitioners also blame undiagnosed gut parasites.

MENTAL ILLNESS

Nutritional factors like food allergy, low blood sugar, deficiencies or even dependencies of B vitamins and zinc, for instance, can result in disturbed behaviour and mental function, such as aggressive outbursts, hallucinations, hyperactivity and depression. However after some years without the appropriate nutritional treatment, ingrained patterns of behaviour may set in, which present a separate problem even though the original problem may have been nutritional.

A nutritional therapist can investigate the possibility of nutritional causes in mental illness and disturbed behaviour, but should ideally work together with a sympathetic psychiatrist.

MIGRAINE

For the nutritional therapist this is one of the easiest illnesses to deal with, and results are often excellent. In our experience food intolerance is without question the most common cause of migraine. A dysfunction involving the conversion of the amino acid cysteine to inorganic sulphate is also thought to be common; this may impair the liver's ability to conjugate xenobiotics in phase II detoxification (see page 67).

MULTIPLE SCLEROSIS

While it is not thought possible to reverse the neurological damage caused by this disease process, many individuals have found that the progress of the disease can be considerably arrested by investigating and treating food intolerances. Tea, coffee and saturated fat seem to be particularly problematic foods for virtually all MS sufferers, and they will also have other allergies which vary from person to person.

PREMENSTRUAL AND MENOPAUSAL PROBLEMS

These are possibly two different sides of the same coin. Premenstrual problems are often easier to deal with than menopausal symptoms, and may be straightforward symptoms of nutritional deficiency, usually involving B vitamins and magnesium, as well as essential fatty acids. One of my patients lost her premenstrual symptoms very shortly after beginning to follow a hypoallergenic diet, but this is relatively rare.

Menopausal symptoms can be difficult to improve, since the nutritional deficiencies have had a longer time period over

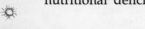

which to inflict their functional damage, and the adrenal glands are thought to be the prime target for this. Nutritional therapists generally aim their treatments at improving adrenal gland function, since healthy adrenals are able to continue making small amounts of oestrogen after the ovaries have stopped production. The pituitary gland will also be a target for treatment, since this is the master gland which controls the adrenals and other parts of the endocrine system.

PROSTATE ENLARGEMENT

Zinc and essential fatty acid deficiencies can encourage prostate enlargement by reducing the formation of prostaglandins which help to control prostate growth. A number of natural remedies, including pollen extracts, the herb Saw palmetto and an amino acid combination have been used successfully in clinical trials to relieve the symptoms of prostate enlargement and sometimes to reduce prostate size.

SKIN AILMENTS

In traditional systems of medicine, the skin is linked with the liver, and therefore any rashes, pimples or discharges from the skin are said to reflect a distressed and overworked liver. Acne, eczema and psoriasis are also linked with deficiencies of vitamin A, zinc, GLA and EPA. Acne is also linked with an excess of saturated fat in the diet, and with intolerances to foods such as chocolate or cocoa and cheese. Eczema is more likely to be linked with common food intolerances.

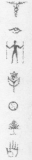

TINNITUS

According to research, a low status of magnesium, B vitamins and essential fatty acids is common in this condition. Fluid retention due to allergies may be a factor, and a toxic overload should be considered. Tinnitus is something which often clears up spontaneously as general health improves while nutritional therapy is being administered for another condition.

11

TOOLS OF NUTRITIONAL THERAPY

Nutritional therapists use a large variety of tools, including different diets, dietary supplements, herbs, and, depending on individual therapists and their training, exercise regimes, stress control techniques, and even so-called 'vibrational' remedies like Bach flower remedies and low-potency homoeopathic remedies. Many nutritional therapists are also trained in other complementary therapies like healing, reflexology and aromatherapy.

DIETARY TOOLS

A nutritional therapist's active treatment diets generally allow only the use of fresh food, unrefined and minimally processed, with care taken to conserve nutrients during cooking, and minimal use of frying.

HYPOALLERGENIC DIET

This is often used as a basic diagnostic diet for the first two weeks of a nutritional therapy regime. It excludes the four foods which are most commonly associated with allergic symptoms (wheat and gluten, dairy produce, eggs and yeast) together with a number of dietary items which may cause actual or potential stress to the digestive system, detoxification system or endocrine system, including tea, coffee and chocolate, sugar, salt, artificial food additives, alcohol, saturated and hydrogenated fat and red meat. The diet is usually given in the form of a checklist of foods to eat and foods to avoid, with suggested recipes and advice on food preparation. In some cases individual guidance for meal planning is also given. This diet must be given under supervision since patients who are faddy eaters have been known to adapt it to taste, and to try to exist on a very small number of foods, quite inadequate for their needs.

Caution: People who have attempted food elimination without proper professional advice often fail to improve for reasons such as not knowing about hidden ingredients in food, not understanding the 'withdrawal' process and so on. If simple eliminations don't work within about two weeks, persistence with self-help is not recommended.

Some practitioners advise their patients to eat only 'rare' foods – foods which the patient has seldom or never eaten before. In this case the diet is known as a 'rare food diet'.

YIN/YANG BALANCED DIETS

These diets are given to individuals whose symptoms suggest an imbalance in yin and yang energies – the energies in the oriental macrobiotic system of medicine which, according to this system, are thought to be at the root of all illness.

Conditions of excess yang are those associated with excessive body heat, inflammations and eruptions. Acne sufferers are often a good example of this. Conditions of excess yang are thought to be much less common than conditions of excess yin in the Western world. Yin conditions are those associated with coldness and lack of energy, chest ailments, and fluid retention. They are thought to be linked with the excess consumption of ice cream, chemicals, drugs and dietary fat and sugar, all of which are considered to be excessively 'yin'.

A diet aiming to reduce excess yang will avoid high-protein foods, and concentrate mainly on brown rice, salad and fresh fruit, vegetables and pulses. A diet aiming to reduce excess yin will avoid raw, cold foods and fruit juices, and concentrate mainly on brown rice, porridge oats, cooked vegetables, miso (a nutritious vegetarian stock paste available from health food shops), pulses and a little cooked fruit and fish.

CLEANSING DIETS (ALKALINIZING DIETS)

There are many variations of cleansing diets, which stem from naturopathic tradition. Often based on raw food, they may not be suitable for people suffering from weakness, or a 'yin' condition of the body, since raw food increases any excess of yin. The main purpose of these diets is to remove excess tissue acidity, a toxic condition caused by the long-term consumption of too much protein, to correct the sodium/potassium balance, to promote cell respiration and oxygenation, and to help decongest the liver after long-term excess fat consumption, and help it to discharge toxic waste matter.

Protein, when metabolized by the body, leaves an acidic residue. This residue may build up in the tissues, causing difficulties in cell oxygenation and, by promoting free radical damage to tissues and joints, may in the long term encourage the development of degenerative diseases such as arthritis and cancers. Research carried out by Professor Louis-Claude Vincent has shown that sufferers of such diseases often have high tissue acidity levels, as shown by measuring urine pH.

Fruits and vegetables, on the other hand, leave an alkaline residue after being metabolized, so cleansing diets mainly concentrate on these, often to the exclusion of all other foods for a short while.

For the first ten days to two weeks cleansing diets are often all raw food. After this some steamed vegetables may be added, and some brown rice and pulses. Some nuts (not peanuts) and a very small amount of olive oil may be allowed, but no other fat. The diet is deliberately low in calories, since it is designed to break up fatty deposits in the liver. Body fats (and lean body tissue) are broken down to release stored energy when calorie intake from food is inadequate for energy needs. To minimize the loss of lean tissue, care must be taken not to reduce the calorie intake too much.

ROTATION DIET

Nutritional therapists use rotation diets for patients with multiple allergies who would not otherwise be able to eat a varied diet. There are many different types of allergic response to foods, and one of these is a type which only occurs if a specific food is eaten more than once in any four-day period. Why four days, and not three or five, for instance, we don't know. Some believe that it takes four days to clear all remains of a food completely out of the system, and that eating it more than once in that period can overload the body's ability to detoxify some of the natural chemicals found in that particular food. It is believed that the rotation diet achieves a gradual regaining of tolerance to foods by reducing an excessive demand for specific liver detoxifying enzymes that are required to metabolize specific natural food toxins. If this demand is not met, and the problem foods continue to be eaten, there may be a rise in circulating toxins or intermediate toxic metabolites, which promotes not only symptoms but biological damage. If the load is reduced, there is an opportunity not only for the enzyme systems in question to regenerate, but also for the biological damage to be repaired.

Each rotation diet must be individually devised according to the patient's own tolerances. The diet will not include foods to which the patient is severely allergic or which always cause an allergic reaction when eaten. Each food in a rotation diet may be eaten only once in any four day-period. Once the patient begins to feel better, this can be modified, and then foods to which the patient has never suffered an allergic reaction need no longer be strictly 'rotated', although they should nevertheless not be eaten too regularly.

FOOD DIARIES

A food diary is not a diet, but it is a useful tool for the nutritional therapist who is trying to identify foods not commonly eaten by a patient, to which that patient does not know that he or she is allergic. Keeping a diary of foods eaten and symptoms experienced will eventually show links, if these exist, between specific foods and symptoms. If a connection between eating and symptoms seems to be definite but links with specific foods seem to be unclear and symptoms seem to occur in a haphazard manner, the therapist will probably take this as a sign of weakness in liver detoxification ability.

FEW FOODS DIET

The 'few foods diet' is a recognized medical technique for identifying food allergens and problem foods, and consists of hospitalizing a patient, starting them off on just a few foods, and then gradually adding more foods, observing which foods seem to set off symptoms when added to the diet. One well known version of the few foods diet is the 'lamb and pears' diet, in which the patient is allowed to eat nothing but lamb and pears for a number of days. Other versions are the 'mackerel and courgettes' diet, or the 'cod and cabbage' diet. In each case the 'few foods' chosen are those considered least likely to provoke an allergic reaction.

It is not advisable to continue with a few foods diet for

more than a few days, and such a diet is only given under the strictest supervision. Although useful for identifying definite allergic reactions which occur within 24 hours, it may not pick up on the more insidious types of allergic response.

FASTING AND MONO DIETS

Fasting is a technique used much more frequently by the more traditional naturopath rather than the modern nutritional therapist. It is based on the theory that if an individual stops eating, the body will have the opportunity to break down and eliminate its diseased parts. Whether or not this is true, fasting certainly enables the digestive system to rest and repair its absorptive ability where impaired (if this is possible and provided dysbiosis is thoroughly treated first).

The most effective type of fast is thought to be the water fast, in which only water is consumed. Also used are juice fasts, in which carrot or apple juice, for instance, may also be consumed, especially after severe diarrhoea, when the body needs to replenish electrolytes and may be unable to tolerate food anyway. 'Mono diets', consisting of eating only one food, like apples or grapes, are also a type of fast.

Water or juice fasts generally last from four days to two weeks. Mono diets may last up to six weeks. Lengthy fasting must only be prescribed and supervised by a knowledgeable practitioner and never self-administered in the hope that it 'might help'. People suffering from any form of weakness are not advised to fast until they are stronger.

LOW CARBOHYDRATE DIET

This is a technique used only as a last resort by nutritional therapists, for patients with a very resistant weight problem that will not respond to a healthy reduced-calorie, high exercise programme. They must be clinically obese, not merely anxious to lose weight for cosmetic reasons. This diet is based on the premise that if you deprive the body of carbohydrate it will have to convert protein and fat into glucose, to obtain the raw energy material it needs. In the process of this conversion there is some calorie wastage.

Although we are not certain that it is this calorie wastage which accounts for the success of this diet, the diet does usually succeed when other diets have failed. However it can lead to acidosis, deydration, loss of lean tissue, and impairment of kidney function due to a build-up of waste products from breakdown of body tissues if used for prolonged periods. Nutritional therapists take great care when administering this diet, and ensure that the patient understands it is a once-only diet, and after the target weight has been reached a healthy lifestyle with strict rationing of high-calorie foods must be permanently maintained so that excessive weight gain never recurs.

THE HAY DIET

This is a modified version of the low carbohydrate diet. One or two meals a day containing carbohydrate are permitted.

The Hay diet has traditionally been promoted as being effective for weight loss and digestive problems because it does not 'mix' starch and protein, thus preventing the body from having to produce starch-digesting and protein-digesting enzymes at the same time. There is no physiological rationale why this enzyme manipulation should help with weight loss. Since a proportion of people do find the Hay diet more effective than a conventional weight-loss diet, this may be because one or two meals a day are low in carbohydrate.

Likewise individuals who do not know that they are allergic to carbohydrate foods such as wheat and rice may also believe it is this enzyme manipulation which helps to relieve their symptoms, not the fact that they are reducing their intake of foods which they do not tolerate well, and which may cause weight gain due to allergic fluid retention. Doubtless weak digestive organs may benefit from not having to produce all types of enzymes for all meals, but the Hay diet is not a permanent solution to a weak digestion, and most nutritional therapists do not often prescribe this rather difficult and complex diet.

THE ANTI-CANDIDA DIET

The anti-Candida diet is intended to discourage the growth of the Candida albicans yeast, described in Chapter 6. Since most candidiasis sufferers have food allergies, the diet is a modified version of the hypoallergenic diet. In addition it does not permit the ingestion of any sweetened foods or any foods or drinks which are very high in natural sugars, such as bananas, fruit juice and dried fruit. This is because sugar encourages the growth of yeasts.

It used to be believed that mushrooms (which are a member of the fungus family), and yeast occurring in stock cubes, yeast extract, baked products, fermented products like soy sauce and vinegar, or even products containing small quantities of these, like mayonnaise, could encourage the growth of the Candida yeast. It is now known that the consumption of killed yeast cannot encourage Candida albicans, and that the aggravation of candidiasis symptoms which was noted by early workers in this field, was almost certainly due to yeast allergy – the candidiasis sufferer having been sensitized to yeast by having a yeast infestation in his or her intestines.

An anti-Candida diet will also encourage the consumption of onions, leeks, extra-virgin olive oil, unsweetened soya yoghurt and garlic, all of which help to inhibit the growth of the yeast.

This diet is famous for its use against cancer, and many so-called anti-cancer diets are variations of it. Dr Max Gerson was a physician practising from the 1930s to the 1950s who invented what was to be a revolutionary but controversial new form of cancer treatment based primarily on the consumption of organically grown fresh, whole foods and large quantities of fruit and vegetable juices, particularly leafy green vegetables. In *A Cancer Therapy: Results of Fifty Cases*, Gerson wrote that cancer is 'a very slow, progressing, imperceptible symptom caused by poisoning of the liver and simultaneously an impairment of the whole intestinal tract'. His treatment therefore aimed to assist liver oxidizing enzymes (now known as cytochrome P450 mixed-function oxidases) and provide extra nourishment in easily-absorbed form (by means of the juices) as well as to enhance the elimination of toxic substances (by means of coffee enemas).

Half a century on, modern science is only now catching up with Max Gerson, as scientists are finding that green vegetables like broccoli and brussels sprouts really do contain powerful substances (indoles) which assist the function of cytochrome P450 oxidase enzymes in the liver. Research also reveals that most cancer patients have some degree of food malabsorption.

BLOOD SUGAR CONTROL DIET

There are two types of blood sugar problem: a tendency to excessively high blood sugar (hyperglycaemia, or diabetes) and a tendency to excessively low blood sugar (hypoglycaemia). Both types are aggravated by the consumption of foods with a high glycaemic index, that is to say foods which are converted very rapidly into blood sugar. Most of these foods can be identified by their sweetness, such as sugar, honey, bananas, fruit juice, carrot juice and dried fruit. Refined starches like white

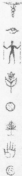

flour and white rice are also more readily converted to sugar than their wholegrain counterparts.

The blood sugar control diet excludes such foods and encourages the use of foods high in soluble fibre like pulses and oatmeal, which help to slow down the absorption of sugars into the bloodstream. It is interesting that orthodox nutritional advice for diabetics has undergone considerable change and is now identical to the advice which nutritional therapists have always given.

MAINTENANCE DIET

A maintenance diet is a diet prescribed for long-term use after a nutritional therapy treatment programme. It aims to keep the individual as healthy as possible, and to prevent their original problem from returning, but with the minimum of inconvenience. Many people first put on a nutritional therapy regime are horrified at their initial, diagnostic diet, believing that they will be asked to eat like this for the rest of their life. Nothing could be further from the truth. There is simply no need for most people to eat a highly restricted diet for lengthy periods of time. Once it has been determined what was contributing to their ill-health, those dietary elements can be omitted, and a more normal diet initiated.

The basic principles of the maintenance diet are that 90 per cent of the diet should consist of a variety of fruit, vegetables, pulses, whole grains or cereals, nuts and seeds daily, and that the remaining 10 per cent can be selected at will, provided that calorie restrictions are observed and allergenic foods avoided. The nutritional therapist will also generally recommend that even if the individual is not allergic to wheat, eggs, yeast and dairy produce, consumption of these foods should be controlled. This is because out of all the foods which form part of the human diet, these seem to be the most highly allergenic, therefore as a species we are probably not well adapted to them and may be well advised to take care with their consumption. It is possible that the genetic engineering to which modern wheat and yeast have been subjected (to make lesser quantities go further in manufactured products) and the antibiotics and/or hormones, food colourings etc, fed to laying hens and dairy cattle, traces of which may remain in eggs and milk, may play some part in this poor adaptation. I am certainly aware that some children who are severely allergic to ordinary dairy milk suffer no reaction to organic milk (milk from cows fed only traditional food and not routinely treated with drugs). Likewise many individuals who are allergic to modern wheat products can tolerate ancient wheat (also known as 'spelt') without problems.

A maintenance diet also requires a restricted intake of tea, coffee, food additives, sugar (including honey), saturated fat and red meat.

The maintenance diet is also suitable for those without health problems who wish to follow healthy eating practices. See Appendix I.

FRUIT AND VEGETABLE JUICES

Fruit and vegetable juices can be powerful aids to nutritional therapy. Because the bulk (fibre) is removed, very large amounts of nutrients can be ingested, and juices can in this sense be described as dietary supplements. Juices can also be used as herbal treatments since some are capable of altering conditions in the body.

Some juice uses: drinking cranberry juice helps to prevent bacteria from adhering to the mucous membrane of the bladder and thus helps to prevent cystitis; celery juice helps to alkalinize the body and acts as a diuretic, being particularly helpful for arthritic conditions; raw cabbage juice contains vitamin U,

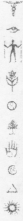

a substance shown in medical trials to help in the healing of peptic ulcers; radish juice is high in organic sulphur, which aids detoxification; and broccoli, cabbage, cauliflower and brussels sprout juices are a rich source of antioxidant nutrients and indoles which aid cytochrome P450 oxidase enzymes in the liver. These help to prevent cancer by detoxifying carcinogens and aid the breakdown of oestrogen. (An excess of oestrogen, caused by inadequate oestrogen breakdown within the body, is a significant factor in the development of breast cancer, fibroids and other female hormone related growths and tumours.)

Juices from leafy green vegetables are rich in chlorophyll, which is capable of neutralizing toxic substances in the gut.

DIETARY SUPPLEMENTS

Dietary supplements are:

1) Preparations of vitamins, minerals, amino acids, essential fatty acids, enzymes, fibre and other factors which fulfil a useful or necessary physiological function and are found in food or synthesized within the body from food. These preparations may be chemically synthesized or natural extracts.

2) Concentrated plant- or animal-source preparations such as fish oils, yeast, probiotics, algae and plant or herb extracts, used to supplement the diet with the nutrients they contain, or for their health-giving properties.

Many books have been published which appear to advocate the use of vitamin and mineral supplements as medicines for specific health problems like PMS, skin diseases, blood sugar problems, fatigue, menopausal symptoms and even cancers. This is for two reasons. First, many experiments were carried out on vitamins soon after their discovery and isolation in the mid-twentieth century, in the hope that they might be able to cure diseases, just as vitamin B_3 was found to cure the mystery disease pellagra. Originally no one knew that pellagra was a vitamin deficiency disease. Likewise they didn't know how many other diseases might be vitamin or mineral deficiency diseases, so there was great interest in this avenue of research until synthetic drugs took over in medical research and changed the fashion completely.

But this means that a great deal of research does exist into the connection between nutrients and specific diseases. Later, as the supplement industry saw the great public interest in this research (stimulated by the writings of authors like Adelle Davis) as a sales opportunity, it encouraged the maximum publicity for any nutrition research which showed beneficial effects for dietary supplementation against diseases. Although it was always likely that these beneficial effects were due to the correction of nutritional deficiencies rather than to any 'medicinal' effect, researchers rarely tested individuals for nutrient status before admitting them into clinical trials. Their rationale was that nutritional deficiencies are extremely rare in the Western world, and therefore any benefits from using large doses of dietary supplements against diseases other than scurvy, beri-beri etc, must be due to a pharmacological (medicine-like) mechanism of action. The industry collaborated in this because it wanted to encourage all sufferers of a particular disease to buy their product.

Clinical trials, usually carried out using single nutrients, frequently showed conflicting results. Some studies would find that there was a positive action against a disease, others would not. This is easily explained by pointing out that only those individuals deficient in these nutrients were likely to benefit

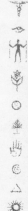

from them. But the net result is that the medical establishment does not take any of these trials seriously, and restricts its use of dietary supplements to low doses used for the routine supplementation of babies' and young children's diets, and for adults in 'risk groups' such as dieters, the elderly and pregnant women, who may not be eating a healthy diet.

DOSAGES

Although in the early days megadoses of nutrients were commonly used, based on experimental dosages in clinical trials, modern nutritional therapy recognizes that equally good if not better results can now be achieved by balancing nutrients – using them with their co-factors and paying attention to product formulation and to other aspects of diet besides supplementation. Now we generally prefer to use dosages in the so-called 'higher range'. This is a range between RDA (Recommended Daily Amount) levels and the megadose ranges still used by conventional doctors in orthodox medicine. (Examples of megadoses used by doctors are 5,000 mcg of vitamin B_{12} in injection form for pernicious anaemia, 4 mg of folic acid for pregnant women, 100 mg iron for pregnant women or anaemia sufferers, 200 mg vitamin B_6 for premenstrual syndrome, or 500 mg vitamin B_3 for high cholesterol.)

The reason for using 'higher range' rather than RDA level supplements is that in our experience symptoms due to nutritional deficiencies are often much more rapidly cleared up with these doses than with smaller amounts.

WHAT FOODS ARE RICH IN . . . ?

There are still a lot of people who, when they see a nutritional therapist and are informed that they may have a zinc deficiency, for example, will ask 'What foods are rich in zinc?' Clearly the question is designed to obtain a list of foods which contain large amounts of the deficient nutrient so that these can be ingested and the deficiency symptoms cured.

It doesn't matter what nutrient the person is asking about, the answer is always the same: 'A varied wholefood diet'. I could, of course, have answered 'oysters', or 'wheatgerm' but this would be misleading. My client might think that by eating a portion of oysters once a week her premenstrual syndrome is going to go away. It won't. With the exception of vitamin A in liver and vitamin D in fish liver oils, there are no foods that are high enough in any particular nutrients to take the place of higher-range supplements. All good foods are balanced sources of many nutrients and the chances are that if you are looking after your diet you are already eating all the right foods. If not, your nutritional therapist will advise you on all-round improvement.

DO YOU NEED TO TAKE SUPPLEMENTS FOR EVER?

As discussed above, dietary supplements are not medicines like blood pressure pills or anti-asthma drugs which have to be taken for ever. They seek to help the body repair the functions which were damaged by the deficiency state, and then you can stop taking them, provided that you continue with your varied wholefood diet. It's a bit like trying to revive a commercial business that's been slowly going bankrupt. You can put some cash back into it to keep things from getting worse, but it's not going to thrive on its own again until you inject a bit of capital so that you can get the machinery and equipment out of hock.

SAFETY

The vitamin industry keeps a keen eye on the scientific literature to ensure that its products are not sold in dosages likely to lead easily to overdose, unless they are deliberately abused.

One survey carried out in the USA by Donald Loomis, reported in the *Townsend Letter for Doctors*, found that dietary supplements were tens of thousands of times less likely than *prescribed* medicines to cause death. And a 1994 study funded by the UK Government into the potential toxic effects of supplements and herbal products found that adverse reactions to vitamins, minerals and traditional Western herbs are extremely rare. This can be compared with the annual admission of an estimated 10,000 people into UK hospitals as a result of adverse reactions to medicines prescribed by their doctors and presumed safe (Social Audit, 1992).

HERBS

The nutritional therapist does not use herbs in the same way as a medical herbalist, who may prescribe them as safer alternatives to orthodox medicines. We use them mainly as diet aids, for instance as follows:

> Golden seal, Artemisia annua, barberry or grapefruit seed extract for their anti-bacterial, anti-fungal and anti-parasitic effects in dysbiotic patients.

> Gentian and other bitter herbs to stimulate the production of gastric acid.

> Comfrey, slippery elm, chamomile and marshmallow to soothe and heal the digestive system after candidiasis or allergic inflammation.

> Dandelion root, turmeric and silymarin to help drain the liver and gall bladder during a detox programme.

Comfrey as a nutritional supplement for people whose bones need strengthening. (Contrary to some information sources, comfrey has not been proved to be a toxic herb. To get cancer from it you would have to eat 27 times your body weight of comfrey leaves.)

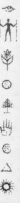

12

ALTERNATIVE
VERSUS ORTHODOX

An indulgent attitude towards a self-indulgent lifestyle is practically endemic in our society. It is the norm to eat food primarily for pleasure. This attitude probably largely stems from the nutrition education of the 1950s, when nutrition was still a very young science and those who 'knew' about it delighted in showing off their sophistication by telling others what tiny amounts of vitamins and minerals the human body needs; how we can eat just about anything we want and not develop deficiencies.

To a large extent this attitude still prevails as far as the setting of government recommended intakes of vitamins and minerals is concerned. In many countries, the Recommended Daily Amount (RDA) for vitamins and minerals can be met by a daily diet consisting of little more than hamburgers, chips, biscuits, half a portion of vegetables and half an apple a day.

Eating the several daily portions of fruit and vegetables now recommended by the World Health Organization would often result in a much larger intake of vitamins and minerals than the RDA level. Yet governments have never adjusted their RDAs accordingly. It doesn't seem logical on the one hand to recommend that for cancer prevention populations should eat large quantities of foods which are very rich in vitamins and minerals, but on the other hand to maintain that a diet containing just a fraction of those amounts is 'adequate to meet the needs of practically the whole population' (the definition of an RDA).

Since orthodox nutritionists usually argue that the RDAs and the food recommendations are not mutually exclusive, and that anyway it's not 'proved' that a diet high in vegetables protects against cancer, let's turn it the other way around. If a catering company supplied schoolchildren or hospital patients with nutrient-rich foods only in the quantity needed to reach their RDA targets, these quantities would be so small that, generally speaking, they would not provide the calories needed for energy purposes. The company would be justified on *scientific* grounds, to make up the extra calories with any cheap junk foods that it pleased: chips, doughnuts, sugary soft drinks and ice cream, for instance. Any further intake of vitamins and minerals would be deemed surplus to requirements.

With so much research around now which points to the micronutrients (vitamins and minerals) in vegetables and fruits as being protective against cancer, it seems deeply irresponsible to maintain that this association is not satisfactorily 'proven' since this will inevitably put people off improving their diet. Social responsibility dictates that any figures for micronutrients which do not match the levels found in the kind of diet now advocated by the World Health Organization, are invalid, and should not be used as a measure of dietary adequacy.

Unfortunately the reverse seems to be happening. In the UK, a new system has been developed for measuring the adequacy of vitamin, mineral and other nutrient intakes in the population as a whole and in meals supplied to institutions. It is likely that other countries will eventually introduce the same system, which has been generally admired in the scientific community. Instead of setting 'recommended' daily amounts, the UK government now seeks to move away from the notion of 'recommendations' by setting 'Dietary Reference Values', consisting of three sets of figures.

The first set of figures is the Reference Nutrient Intake (RNI) which represents the amount of a nutrient that is deemed sufficient to meet the needs of practically all healthy people – even those with higher than normal needs. As the table shows, it is roughly equivalent to the old RDA.

Next we have the Estimated Average Requirement (EAR) which represents the amount of a nutrient that is sufficient to meet the needs of the average individual. Dietitians are taught that if a group of people are consuming these levels of nutrients, they are unlikely to develop nutritional deficiencies. According to a spokesperson for the British Dietetic Association, meals in institutions will, generally speaking, be considered adequate if they achieve vitamin and mineral levels between the RNI and the EAR.

Finally we have the Lower Reference Nutrient Intake (LRNI) which represents an amount of a nutrient that is virtually certain to be inadequate. (The average intake of the trace element selenium in the UK falls well below this figure).

Nutrients	Old RDA	RNI*	EAR*	LRNI*	Minimum WHO diet contains
			Given as daily amounts		
Vitamin A	750mcg	700mcg	500mcg	300mcg	399mcg
Thiamin	1.2mg**	1.0mg	0.3mg	0.23mg	1.2mg
Riboflavin	1.6mg	1.3mg	1.0mg	0.8mg	1.4mg
Niacin	18mg	17mg	5.5mg	4.4mg	27.1mg
Vitamin B6	-	1.4mg†	1.2mg†	1.0mg†	1.7mg
Vitamin B12	-	1.5mcg	1.25mg	1.0mcg	1.0mcg
Folate	-	200mcg	150mcg	100mcg	233mcg
Vitamin C	30mg	40mg	25mg	10mg	89.4mg
Vitamin D	-	-	-	-	1.9mcg
Vitamin E	-	-	-	-	-
Calcium	500mg	750mg	525mg	400mg	1,100mg
Phosphorus	-	550mg	400mg	310mg	1,202mg
Magnesium	-	300mg	250mg	190mg	358mg
Sodium	-	1,600mg	-	575mg	-
Potassium	-	3,500mg	-	2,000mg	3,948mg
Chloride	-	2,500mg	-	885mg	-
Iron	10mg	8.7mg	6.7mg	4.7mg	12.2mg
Zinc	-	9.5mg	7.3mg	5.5mg	6.62mg
Copper	-	1.2mg	-	-	2.09mg
Selenium	-	75mcg	-	40mcg	-
Iodine	-	140mcg	-	70mcg	-
Calories			2,550Kcal		1,920Kcal

* These are the figures for males aged 19-50 years

** This is the figure for moderately active young men

† Based on a daily protein intake of 14.7% of total energy (calories)

Comparison of former RDA and new Dietary Reference Values, with a random sample diet designed by the Food Commission to meet the minimum recommendations for disease prevention, of the World Health Organisation. (Reprinted from *Nutritional Therapy Today*, March 1992, Society for the Promotion of Nutritional Therapy, UK).

UK Dietary Reference Values compared with values found in a diet meeting WHO standards

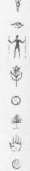

PRINCIPLES OF NUTRITIONAL THERAPY

These dietary reference values are much vaunted as 'Scientifically Correct'.

The alternative nutrition movement blames the meddling of science for many of today's ills. The food industry in particularly uses 'Scientific Correctness' to deliberately obscure common sense judgments about food matters. Those who warn of the dangers of excessive consumption of its refined and nutrient-depleted products are mockingly asked to provide 'scientific proof' of such dangers. But the 'scientific proof' is strangely never good enough. A clever scientist can run rings around the advocates of healthy eating with arguments about what constitutes 'proper' proof. To those in the know, it is a game. The media, who don't know the rules of the game, are often bamboozled and confused to the extent that articles on wholefood eating and the use of vitamin supplements are relegated by editors to women's pages and light magazines, not published as serious news articles or reports.

The food industry is extremely powerful and influential in government circles, universities and other teaching establishments, hospitals and research institutions. Like the drug industry, it gives research grants to encourage institutions not to do or say anything which it might disagree with, and may even put its own employees in influential positions within these institutions. Leading academics who are not widely known to be in the industry's pay may be trotted out from time to time to make highly publicized announcements that such and such an item of junk food is 'highly nutritious'. Such announcements are 'Scientifically Correct'. Fat is a nutrient, therefore any food high in fat can accurately be described as highly nutritious even if the words mean something entirely different to the average lay person.

The industry also distributes promotional literature to doctors' surgeries in the guise of health advice. When I worked for a GP I was surrounded with stacks of 'patients' advice' leaflets that had never been ordered nor asked for, urging people to eat butter and meat. Naturally the sole purpose of these leaflets was to give these foods a healthier image after cholesterol and BSE scare stories in the media had damaged sales. Most people will believe that if they obtained a leaflet from a doctor's surgery then the leaflet's authority is equivalent to a doctor's authority.

Scientific Correctness can also have tragic consequences. In the early 1980s research was carried out by Professor Richard Smithells in the UK into the role of vitamin deficiencies in spina bifida and other birth defects known as neural tube defects, where the foetus' nervous system does not develop properly. This leads to deformity or major disability such as total absence of the skull, defective brain development or absence of the brain and spinal cord, leading to death. This research showed a clear link between spina bifida and a deficiency of the B vitamin known as folic acid or folate. But no announcement was made by the UK government that all women anticipating pregnancy should ensure an adequate intake of folic acid from green vegetables and orange juice. Doctors were not instructed to give this advice. What did the government do instead? It withdrew the RDA for folic acid. Since RDAs were only published for nutrients considered to be at risk of deficiency, the non-publication of an RDA for folic acid was tantamount to a statement by the scientific community that folic acid was not likely to be in short supply in anyone's diet.

This is one of the most horrific scandals of the twentieth century, resulting in thousands of cases of spina bifida which could so easily have been prevented. In the mid-1970s, before spina bifida was routinely detected during pregnancy and women offered abortions, the incidence was one in 100 births in Scotland, Wales and Ireland.

Despite Professor Smithells' work, the scientists' rationale for their decision to abolish the RDA was that there was no 'proof' of a link between folic acid deficiency and such birth defects.

How can the phrase 'there is no proof' ever be trusted again? Ten years and many more trials later the link was suddenly considered acceptable after all and announcements were made that folic acid consumption should be increased. But why so reluctantly? Whatever excuse can be fabricated, it will not be adequate. What a woman at risk of giving birth to a deformed baby wants is information that could help her. She is not interested in the intricacies of scientific correctness and what constitutes 'proof' to the trained scientific mind, safely detached from the rest of the human race in its academic closet. In most people's opinion Professor Smithells' early work would have constituted very adequate proof if their own family was at stake.

With monotonous regularity we hear orthodox nutritionists telling us that 'there is no evidence' or 'no proof' of this or that principle of alternative nutrition or nutritional therapy. When you tell them about the research on which that principle is based, or point out its biochemical rationale, you will almost always meet with resistance, hostility or evasive answers. Of course no one likes to be told how to do their job, or to have their most cherished beliefs challenged, but if the people who are officially in charge of our health do not provide a satisfactory service, then the public will turn elsewhere.

The dietetic profession is keenly aware of the public's interest in alternative nutritional therapy, and attempts have been made in some states of the USA to make it illegal to give nutritional advice without a conventional dietetics diploma. In the UK the media have unwittingly been used as a propaganda tool to turn the public away from alternative nutritional therapists by claiming that they are incompetent, potentially dangerous and improperly trained.

Those who are working to get complementary medicine and nutritional therapy more widely accepted need the support of those they have helped. Write to your doctor explaining how you got well. Write to the local health authority, to local government health departments and to your Member of Parliament or Congressman. Tell them your story. Tell them that doctors need to refer their patients to nutritional therapists and other complementary medicine practitioners, and to employ them in their practices. If everybody does this, the sheer weight of numbers will force change in this modern consumer society. What the consumer wants, the consumer gets. Invite orthodox doctors and nutritionists to come out into the free-thinking world and discover through their own experience that the new nutrition is the key to preventing and treating many of today's most devastating diseases.

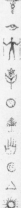

THE
MAINTENANCE DIET

This diet is used for general healthy eating purposes and after the completion of an active nutritional therapy programme.

Eat foods from the above groups in the proportions shown. You may also select other foods of your own choice in proportion to the size of the 'Free Choice' panel. The secret of avoiding deficiencies is to ensure the daily consumption of a good variety of foods from each group and not to become dependent on a small range of foods.

IMPORTANT

If you do not eat fish or poultry regularly, and if you have cut read meat, eggs and dairy produce down to very low levels or do not eat them at all, then you should ensure that you eat a selection every day of the vegetables, complex carbohydrates and other foods listed in the pyramid in italics.

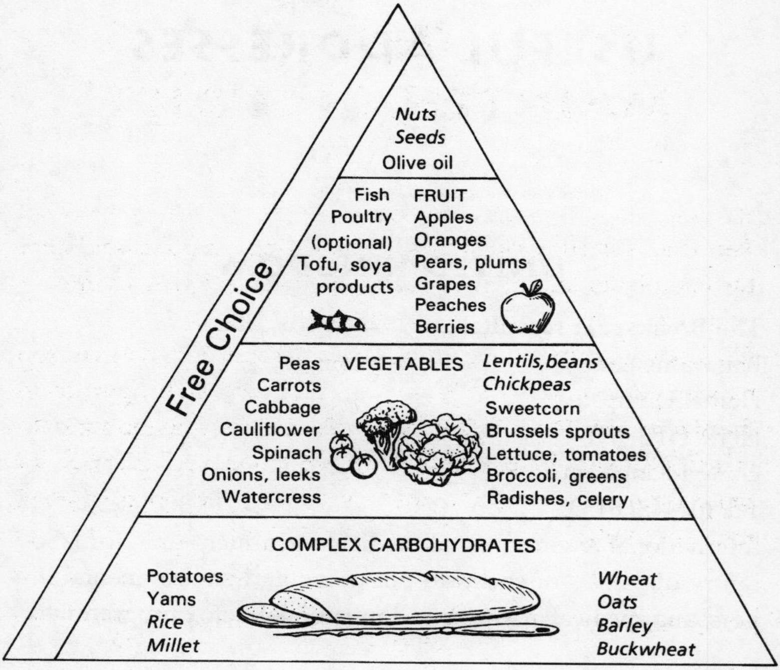
Nuts
Seeds
Olive oil
Fish
Poultry
(optional)
Tofu, soya
products
FRUIT
Apples
Oranges
Pears, plums
Grapes
Peaches
Berries
Free Choice
Peas
Carrots
Cabbage
Cauliflower
Spinach
Onions, leeks
Watercress
VEGETABLES
Lentils, beans
Chickpeas
Sweetcorn
Brussels sprouts
Lettuce, tomatoes
Broccoli, greens
Radishes, celery
COMPLEX CARBOHYDRATES
Potatoes
Yams
Rice
Millet
Wheat
Oats
Barley
Buckwheat

USEFUL ADDRESSES

UNITED KINGDOM

The Breakspear Hospital
Belswains Lane
Hemel Hempstead
Herts HP3 9HP
United Kingdom
Tel: (01442) 61333
International environmental medicine treatment unit, for laboratory diagnosis of chemical poisoning and environmental illness, and medically supervised nutritional detox programmes.

Bristol Cancer Help Centre
Grove House
Cornwallis Grove
Clifton
Bristol BS8 4PG
United Kingdom
Tel: (0117) 974 3216
A residential and day centre for cancer patients who wish to learn about holistic approaches to cancer care.

British Society for Mercury-Free Dentistry
1 Welbeck House
62 Welbeck St
London W1M 7HB
United Kingdom
Send SAE for a register of UK mercury-free dentists.

British Hypnosis Research Register
8 Paston Place
Brighton
East Sussex BN2 1HA
United Kingdom
Tel: (01273) 693622
Register of Eriksonian hypnotherapists. Ask for a copy of the register.

British Society for Allergy and Environmental Medicine
PO Box 28
Totton
Southampton
Hants SO40 2ZA
United Kingdom
A society of doctors who recognize the broad principles of nutritional therapy as described in this book and treat patients accordingly.

Centre for Autogenic Training
100 Harley Street
London W1N 1AF
United Kingdom
Tel: (0171) 935 1811
Contact the Centre for information on autogenic training and local centres which provide it.

Community Health Foundation
188 Old Street
London EC1V 9BP
United Kingdom
Tel: (0171) 251 4076
International centre for training in oriental nutritional therapy (macrobiotics).

Eating Disorders Association
Sackville Place
44 Magdalen St
Norwich
Norfolk NR3 1JE
United Kingdom
Tel: (01603) 621414
Provides help and guidance for those with eating disorders.

Foresight (the Association for Preconceptional Care)
28 The Paddock
Godalming
Surrey GU7 1XD
United Kingdom
Tel: (01483) 427839

International Federation of Practitioners of Natural Therapeutics
46 Pulens Crescent
Sheet
Petersfield
Hants GU31 4DH
United Kingdom
Tel: (01730) 266790
International naturopathy umbrella body.

MEDesign Ltd
Clock Tower Works
Railway St
Southport
Merseyside PR8 5BB
United Kingdom
Tel: (01704) 542373
Phone to find nearest Back Friend stockist.

Society for the Promotion of Nutritional Therapy
PO Box 47
Heathfield
East Sussex TN21 8ZX
United Kingdom
Tel: (01435) 867007
Email and Internet: 100045.255@compuserve.com.
Registration body for nutritional therapists. Also educational and campaigning organization with branches throughout the UK and members in many foreign countries. Publishes educational magazine *Nutritional Therapy Today* for members. Factsheets and other publications also available.

Send £1 for information on nutritional therapy, membership of the society and a list of your nearest practitioners.

American Academy of Environmental Medicine
4510 W. 89th Street
Prairie Village
Kansas 66207
USA
Tel: (913) 341 3625
Register of practitioners of environmental medicine.

American Environmental Health Foundation
8345 Walnut Hill Lane
Suite 200
Dallas
Texas 75231–4262
USA
Tel: (214) 368 4132
Organization for the recognition and appropriate treatment of environmental illness. Books and publications available.

American Preventive Medical Association
275 Millway
PO Box 732
Barnstable
ME 02630
USA
Tel: (508) 362 4343
Register of practitioners sympathetic to a natural approach to medicine.

Citizens for Health
PO Box 1195
Tacoma
WA 98401
USA
Tel: (206) 922 2457
Campaigns for consumer rights in natural medicine.

Linus Pauling Institute
440 Page Mill Road
Palo Alto
CA 94306–2031
USA
Tel: (415) 327 4064
Centre for research into vitamin C.

AUSTRALIA

**Australian College of Nutritional & Environmental
Medicine**
13 Hilton St
Beaumaris
Victoria 3193
Australia
Tel: 9589 6088
For a referral service for all conventionally trained GPs and
specialists who are interested in a wider and more natural
approach to illness.

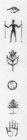

Australian Natural Therapists Association
Taren Point
PO Box 2517
Sydney 2232
Australia

CANADA

Society for Orthomolecular Medicine
16 Florence Avenue
Toronto
Canada M2N 1E9
Tel: (416) 733 2117

NEW ZEALAND

Association of Natural Therapies
81 Forrest Hill Road
Milford
Auckland
New Zealand

New Zealand Natural Health Practitioners Accreditation Board
PO Box 37–491 Auckland
New Zealand
Society of Naturopaths

Box 19183 Auckland 7

New Zealand

INDEX

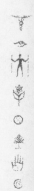

In the same series...

PRINCIPLES OF HYPNOTHERAPY

VERA PEIFFER

Interest in hypnotherapy has grown rapidly over the last few years. Many people are realizing that it is an effective way to solve problems such as mental and emotional trauma, anxiety, depression, phobias and confidence problems, and eliminate unwanted habits such as smoking. This introductory guide explains:

- what hypnotherapy is
- how it works
- what its origins are
- what to expect when you go for treatment
- how to find a reputable hypnotherapist

Vera Peiffer is a leading authority on hypnotherapy. She is a psychologist in private practice in West London specializing in analytical hypnotherapy and a member of the Corporation of Advanced Hypnotherapy.

PRINCIPLES OF SELF-HEALING

DAVID LAWSON

In these high pressure times we are in need of ways of relaxing and gaining a sense of happiness and peace. There are many skills and techniques that we can master to bring healing and well-being to our minds and bodies.

This introductory guide includes:

- visualizations to encourage our natural healing process

- affirmations to guide and inspire

- ways of developing the latent power of the mind

- techniques for gaining a deeper understanding of yourself and others

David Lawson is a teacher, healer and writer. He has worked extensively with Louise Hay, author of *You Can Heal Your Life*, and runs workshops throughout the world. He is the author of several books on the subject, including *I See Myself in Perfect Health*, also published by Thorsons.

PRINCIPLES OF COLONIC IRRIGATION

JILLIE COLLINGS

The popularity of colonic irrigation – the flushing out of the colon to reduce the deposits building up on its walls – has grown steadily over the last few years. Many people are finding the treatment highly effective in ridding the body of toxins, thought to affect both mental and physical function.

This introductory guide explains:

- what colonic irrigation is
- how it works
- what happens during a treatment
- how it can benefit sufferers of constipation and other disorders

Jillie Collings is a successful author and investigative journalist specializing in health issues.